MAMASTE

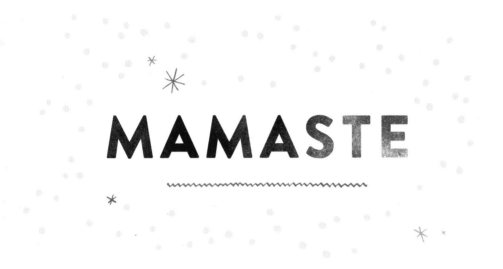

MAMASTE

Discover a More Authentic, Balanced, and
Joyful Motherhood from Within

Lori Bregman

WITH Ursula Cary

CHRONICLE BOOKS

SAN FRANCISCO

Library of Congress Cataloging-in-Publication Data:

Names: Bregman, Lori, author. | Cary, Ursula, author.
Title: Mamaste / Lori Bregman with Ursula Cary.
Description: San Francisco : Chronicle Books, 2018.
Identifiers: LCCN 2018016480 | ISBN 9781452169569 (pbk. : alk. paper)
Subjects: LCSH: Motherhood. | Motherhood—Religious aspects.
Classification: LCC HQ759 .B757 2018 | DDC 306.874/3—dc23
LC record available at https://lccn.loc.gov/2018016480

Manufactured in China

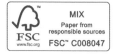

Design by Cat Grishaver

10 9 8 7 6 5 4 3 2 1

Chronicle books and gifts are available at special quantity discounts to
corporations, professional associations, literacy programs, and other
organizations. For details and discount information, please contact our
corporate/premiums department at corporatesales@chroniclebooks.com
or at 1-800-759-0190.

Chronicle Books LLC
680 Second Street
San Francisco, California 94107
www.chroniclebooks.com

*The mother within me
honors the mother within you
because I am you and you are me.
When you are in this place in you
and I am in this place in me,
we are one.*

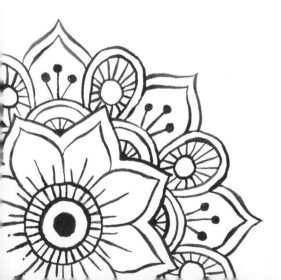

CONTENTS

I believe it is absolutely
possible for all of us
to live authentically
and get along without
judgment or negativity.

*

It's all about taking that one moment to stop and create a little space to coexist and remind ourselves that we are more alike than different.

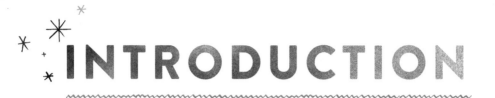

INTRODUCTION

The mother within me honors the mother within you because I am you and you are me. When you are in this place in you and I am in this place in me, we are one. Living the *Mamaste* way helps us live with less judgment and separateness by embracing more compassion and acceptance because we realize that we are each other.

As a doula and in my practice as a wellness/life coach for moms-to-be and new moms, I've worked with all types of women. I build strong relationships with my clients by getting to know them individually and then tailoring our conversations and exercises to fit their specific needs. My goal is always to empower my clients to stay true to who they are, and help them make choices that are right for them—not for anyone else! This may sound simple, but trust me, it's not. Pregnancy and motherhood can do a number on anyone's self-esteem and intuition, and every decision or action can chip away at your confidence, further disconnecting you from your own truth.

Whether they are trying to get pregnant, have a baby on the way, or are seasoned mothers, no two women, children, couples, or families are ever the same. One of the things that makes me good at what I do (and why I love my job!) is that I build a deep relationship with each of my clients. I really get to know and understand the way they operate, and I adjust my approach accordingly. I bring in unique tools to support each person individually and help them discover their own unique gifts and challenges.

It was through this customized work with clients that I observed the commonalities we all possess. I saw the same five expressions appear again and again, albeit at different times and in different ways. Some women are clearly dominant in one type of expression while others balance between two, and, less often, some move comfortably among all five, depending on what life is calling for them at that moment. Once I realized the same five expressions were present in everyone, I was excited to capture my discoveries in a book to share with *all* moms—not just those I have the privilege of working with one-on-one.

Years ago one of my therapists taught me something that stayed with me. She said that it's often what we don't like or are triggered by in another that is what we don't like or accept within ourselves. This hit home for me and became one of the core principles of *Mamaste*. When you feel triggered by someone else's behavior, pause and ask yourself: *What are they reflecting back to me? Is it something I don't like, or a part of myself I am not comfortable with?* If you're constantly judging others or are on the defensive, you may miss this moment of reflection. But if you can accept that we all share the same expressions, we just express them differently, then you'll see that we can learn so much about ourselves from each other. *The mother in me honors the mother in you.*

The mom world is full of judgment, shaming, comparison, envy, and jealousy—and I am willing to bet that you've experienced all or some of these or participated in some small way.

The one thing I know for sure is that all mamas struggle with motherhood in one way or another. No one is immune. Let's face it: motherhood is hard enough without adding to the negativity. What if you chose empathy instead of judgment? What if you saw others as a mirror for yourself? Not to compare, but to ask, how am I like this, too? There's no doubt that it takes courage and self-awareness to acknowledge that truth.

Mamaste is also about reflecting within yourself. Many of my clients reach out to me postpartum for coaching. They say that they don't feel like themselves anymore, and I tell them it's because they aren't the same person they were before. Pregnancy and birth are incredibly powerful, transformative experiences, and for many women, their primary expression shifts to something new and unexpected. This can be confusing, frustrating, or even scary. Integrating new expressions can bring out feelings that have been repressed for years, even decades. Even just by reading through this book and understanding the depth of each expression, you'll be better prepared to recognize internal shifts and use these tools to work through any uncertain moments.

My client Rasha[1] was a dominant Action Mama. As her doula, I watched her plan and organize everything throughout her pregnancy. Three months before her due date, she had already installed the car seat and packed her hospital bag. After she gave birth to her son, she became super laid-back and let go of her need to manage everything. None of the things she had meticulously arranged seemed important anymore. Her primary expression had shifted to Flow Mama. Rasha liked this new mode, but

1 Some names have been changed to protect the privacy of individuals.

she didn't feel "normal," which made her uncomfortable. She kept comparing herself to how she had been before the birth. I asked what her attachment to Action was, and she said, "I'm not achieving anything or getting anywhere." I then asked her to reflect on what she was doing right now with her child. Rasha realized that being a parent actually requires a whole lot of DOING! It was just on another scale from what she was used to. She allowed herself to integrate and enjoy balancing her new normal.

Embracing *Mamaste* can work in big or small ways. From tackling deep-seated fears to letting go of your "ideal" self, you'll be able to access each expression and let it serve you as needed. When your mind starts spinning and you feel like pointing fingers, you'll remember to pause and take a breath: *Mamaste.* When you do this, the negativity stops immediately because you've acknowledged that you're part of the universal motherhood. You're part of a tribe that needs more kindness, love, and light in order to shine a path forward for our children.

This innovative concept brings a unique consciousness to motherhood, and I am inspired to share it with you. I have been deeply blessed to work so intimately with all kinds of amazing women, and in this process they have taught me so much. They have shared with me their collective experiences and invaluable perspective. I've learned that birds of a feather do flock together, but opposites can attract. And how much richer are our lives when we invite those in who are not like us? Integrating new expressions creates greater harmony and balance, and is often the secret to finding that elusive, authentic inner joy and peace we all seek.

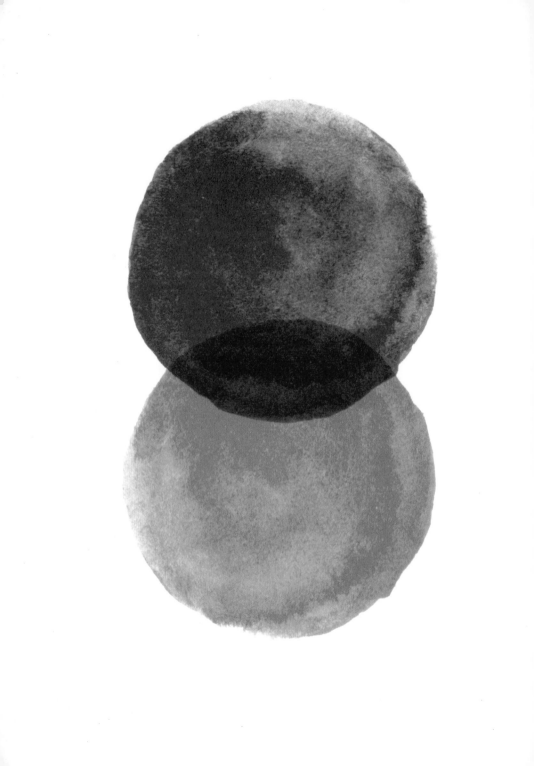

chapter one

THE PATH TO MAMASTE

〰〰〰〰〰〰〰〰〰〰〰〰

This is not a book about breastfeeding versus formula, sleep training versus co-sleeping, or working mamas versus stay-at-home mamas. This is a book for any mom, or anyone with mamas in their life (and by the way, all women can serve as mothers, too). It's a guide to better understanding yourself, to finding more harmony and balance within, and to engaging positively in the fraught mommy world.

Of course, we're all unique, but I've narrowed my focus down to five expressions of motherhood: Action, Flow, Rebel, Vulnerable, and Free. We'll get into what they all mean soon enough, but for now, just know that we *all* possess *all* five expressions. That's right. *Mamaste* means, quite simply, *The mother in me honors the mother in you.* If I am you and you are me, then we must share each other's strengths and weaknesses. We must be more alike than different (after you read this book you will see that we truly are). And if we're mostly the same, then why don't we understand each other? Why do we often seek to tear each other down instead of rising up together to support one another?

Once you realize that you embody all five expressions of motherhood, you won't be able to judge that mom who does things so differently, because in fact, there is an aspect of that mom in you! You may each embody the same expression very uniquely—your vulnerability may not look like hers, but I'm sure you have both experienced moments of fear. Understanding and accepting all five expressions within yourself is the biggest first step; making peace with the expressions that you're uncomfortable with is the next step. This book will help you do both and, most importantly, integrate the expressions in various ways that are truly authentic to you.

Motherhood often strips away some of the expressions you think you're tied to and opens up a whole new outlook. As I wrote in *The Mindful Mom to Be*, you're not only giving birth to a baby, you're giving birth to yourself as a mother. It's an incredible (and sometimes incredibly challenging) transformation that begs for openness, acceptance, and empathy. At any stage in your life, you may relate more strongly to one expression or another.

We all have these different parts of ourselves that I am calling expressions (some like to use the term *archetypes*). Some of these expressions are more active and present, and others lie dormant or repressed. I first experienced this years ago when I worked with a healer. He was doing an energy session with me and after an hour he asked me to do some breath work. I started breathing and this feeling as if I wanted to cry came up so clearly. I looked him in the eye and said, in the strangest, innocent, little-girl voice, "I want to cry."

"Let her out," he said, and I reverted back to my normal (Rebel) internal voice: *No, no, I'm okay.* We did some more breathing exercises, and he asked me to make eye contact as I breathed.

He repeated, "Let her out." And I said again in that vulnerable childlike voice, "I'm so scared." *Where was this coming from?!* I felt really uncomfortable, as if I was having some sort of psychotic episode! The healer reassured me that he was helping to pull out my inner child, the vulnerable self that I had long ago repressed deep down inside.

Later, when I assisted Deborah Raoult in her Birthing from Within class, I heard her tell the group that all their different archetypes (or expressions) would most likely come out at some point in labor and birth. They all make up who you are and will be part of your birthing journey as well as your entire journey of life.

When my co-writer, Ursula, gave birth to her daughter, Zoe, she admitted, "I thought I'd want to control everything like a true Action Mama. I even sent out a detailed email letting my family know when they could visit the hospital! But once the baby was born, I felt my mind and heart shifting away from rigidity and more toward Flow. I just wanted to enjoy the quiet moments with my baby and not worry about all the details." As Ursula navigated her new role, she noticed other shifts, too. "I tend to avoid conflict, and 99 percent of the time I'm willing to go along with others' preferences. But sometimes I feel railroaded into going along with things that don't feel right. Having a baby has helped me channel my inner Rebel and stand firm for what I need or believe in. In my own way, I can say 'no' until my voice is heard."

You may relate to the idea that the things we resist are the things we need to tap into the most. When I feel irritated or triggered by another person, I always know it's because they're expressing something I really need to pay attention to, accept, or heal within myself. Often what we dislike in another is part of our own self-criticism, or a repressed part of ourselves that we work really hard to keep beneath the surface. That's a lot of energy spent fighting your own being! By experiencing and channeling all five expressions, you'll build deeper self-awareness and let your whole self exist. This amazing, radical kind of honesty and awareness is how we grow strong enough to practice empathy not just with ourselves, but for others, too. *Mamaste* is the path to the elusive inner peace as well as peace in the world, which we all crave so much.

Moms today face a constant stream of information, choices, activities, and pressures like never before. You're bombarded with ads and social media feeds, mommy chat rooms and lengthy blog posts on how to pack the perfect lunch, preschool rules and complicated schedules. And that's not even including the seemingly endless daily tasks (naps, meals, diaper changes, colic, messes, LOADS OF LAUNDRY, tantrums, sick days, sleep training, potty training) of *actually* taking care of your kids! As a doula, I help moms-to-be make the right choices and advocate for themselves throughout their pregnancies. As a life/wellness coach, I help moms use all five expressions to work toward a deeper self-awareness and navigate their own set of choices. The mom world is hard enough! Let's make a shift away from fear and judgment. Let's seek harmony both with others and within.

Let's agree to come together, if not for our own health and sanity, then for our kids. I've been incredibly privileged to witness the magic of birth many, many times, and then see those beautiful babies grow and blossom into extraordinary individuals. As I continue to work with clients and friends as they transition into motherhood, I've come to understand how much children really do watch, mimic, and become. In today's world, where hate runs rampant and has the power to separate and divide us all, we must seek love and kindness as our bridge over the madness. It's up to us, as mothers, aunties, friends, and *women*, to be the role models for our children and give them a path to greatness for the future, because the future is in their hands.

Within these pages, you'll discover your own path to *Mamaste* using a variety of helpful tools and information. First, you'll take the quiz in chapter 2, which will help you identify your primary expression, as well as how the other expressions manifest together within you. Then, as you read about each expression, you'll find useful tools and relatable anecdotes to better understand and appreciate your inner self. I've created special mindfulness exercises, journal work, and prompts to help you deepen your self-awareness.

DISCLAIMER: Please note, some of the advice in this book (yoga, essential oils) is not specifically recommended for pregnant women. If you are pregnant, please consult your caregiver before performing any physical activities or using topical oils.

Contributors

I've tapped a wonderfully talented group of friends and colleagues who have provided the ultimate toolkit for each expression, offering a range of resources from essential oils and crystals to yoga sequences and meditations, designed to help you find balance, harmony, and inner peace. I'm thrilled to share their expertise with you! Your team includes:

✳ *Heather Askinosie* is a leading influencer on the power of crystals, feng shui, and holistic healing, with more than twenty-five years of experience studying with the best international healers. In 2000, Heather cofounded Energy Muse, a conscious lifestyle brand, and published a book, *Crystal Muse*, providing tools of empowerment, inspiration, and hope in the tangible form of jewelry and crystals. Here she offers customized crystal recommendations, tailored to the unique needs and energies of each expression. Visit Heather at energymuse.com.

✳ *Lena George* is a certified hypnotherapist, holistic nutritionist, and advanced EFT/Tapping instructor. She teaches weekly classes at Unplug Meditation in Los Angeles and works privately either in person or via Skype. For this book she created an exercise specifically for Free Mamas called Acupressure for the Emotions on page 178. Visit her at lena-george.com.

✳ **MaryRuth Ghiyam** is a certified health educator, nutrition consultant, and chef, who has worked with private clients for more than a decade. She is also the founder of an organic and gluten-free product line called MaryRuth Organics that includes the number-one-selling liquid vitamin in the nation. She contributes a list of important natural remedies for the Vulnerable Mama on page 148. You can visit her at maryruthorganics.com.

✳ **Alessandro Giannetti** is an intuitive and spiritual teacher and founder of the School of Guided Light Healing, which he started to help people reach their highest spiritual potentials. Alessandro shares his Human Pendulum exercise on page 77, which can help all mamas trust their inner voice and make the choices that are right for them. Visit him at guidedlighthealing.com.

✳ **Elissa Goodman** is a holistic nutritionist, a lifestyle cleanse expert, and the author of *Cancer Hacks* (she is a survivor of Hodgkin's lymphoma). The creator of Cleanse Your Body, Cleanse Your Life and the S.O.U.P. Cleanse, she is a certified integrative nutritionist from the American University of Complementary Medicine. She holds a BS in advertising and marketing from Arizona State and a BS in business from the University of Arizona. Elissa has provided nutritional supplement recommendations tailored specifically for each mama expression. Visit her at elissagoodman.com.

✳ **Michele Meiche** is an intuitive soul coach, the author of *Meditation for Everyday Living*, and the host and executive producer of the podcast *Awakenings*. She has generously provided customized meditations for each mama expression, guiding you step-by-step through imagery and mantras to feel more connected and empowered. Visit her at soulplayground.com.

✳ **Heng Ou** is the founder of MotherBees dishes and drinks, inspired by the healing foods she experienced during her own regimen of *zuo yuezi*, the Chinese tradition of postpartum care. Her recipes combine traditional Eastern and Western ingredients to fortify the body after pregnancy and birth, encourage lactation, and calm hormones. Heng is also the author of *The First Forty Days: The Art of Nourishing the New Mother*. You'll find handcrafted recipes for each mama expression that are both healing and delicious. Visit her at motherbees.com.

✳ **Dr. Habib Sadeghi** is the founder of Be Hive of Healing Integrative Medical Center in Agoura Hills, California, specializing in comprehensive and holistic treatment protocols for chronic illnesses. He has served as an attending physician at UCLA Santa Monica Medical Center and is currently a clinical instructor of family medicine at Western University of Health Sciences. He also holds a master's degree in spiritual psychology from the University of Santa Monica and is the author of *Within* and *The Clarity Cleanse.* In this book he shares his groundbreaking PEW-12 exercise on page 139, which has helped clear the minds of many of my clients (and myself!). Visit Dr. Sadeghi at behiveofhealing.com.

✳ **Martha Soffer** is an internationally acclaimed Ayurvedic Panchakarma expert, Ayurvedic chef, herbal Rasayanist, master Ayurvedic pulse diagnostician, and the founder of the renowned Surya Spa. Together with Aleiela Quintero-Allen, an Ayurvedic Panchakarma therapist and a birth and postpartum doula, she has created an Ayurvedic practice specifically geared toward the Flow Mama on page 71. Visit Martha and Aleiela at suryaspa.com.

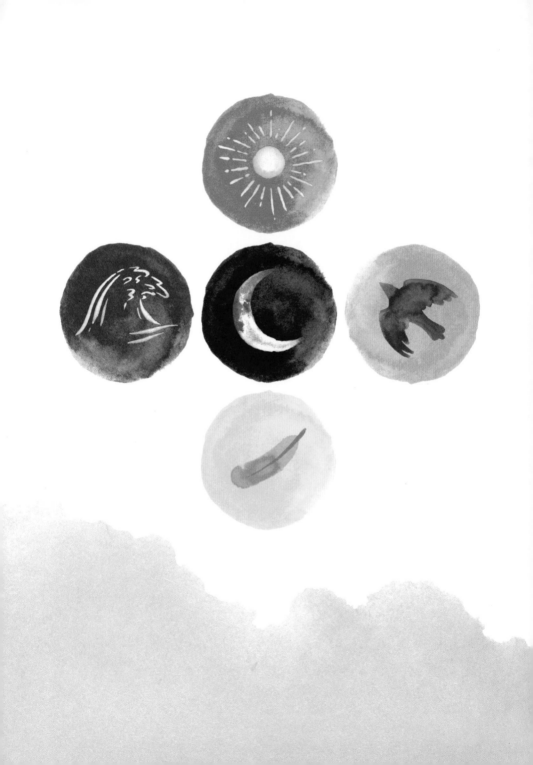

chapter two

THE FIVE EXPRESSIONS OF MOTHERHOOD

So, you might be wondering,
what kind of mom am I?!

Remember, this approach is not meant to corner you into any one "type" or make you feel as if only one part of this book will be useful to you. Rather, it will show you how ALL five mama expressions manifest in you so that you can focus where you need to. This assessment will help you identify your primary mama expression along with a breakdown of the other expressions that we *all* embody. It will help you better understand how each expression manifests within you, and how you can channel them to practice greater understanding and compassion for more balance and harmony within.

As I wrote this book, I identified strongly as Rebel, followed by a tie of Free/Flow, then Action, and finally, Vulnerable. This didn't surprise me, as following the norm has never been my thing. I have a lot to learn from all the expressions, but I know the one I struggle with the most is Vulnerable. I have a hard time asking for help, expressing my needs, or sharing my emotions with others. But I have to embrace my vulnerabilities, not only to seek help when I need it, but to be there for others in their time of need with real empathy and compassion. There is that saying, *You can't love another until you truly love yourself*. You can't be there or accept another until you embrace and accept what's within you. By focusing on the expression that showed up as the "lowest" score, I'm actually uncovering the part of me that needs the most attention. Without integrating this aspect of myself back in, I will continue to live out of balance.

My co-writer, Ursula, easily identified as Action, then Flow— and then Vulnerable, something she didn't expect. "That was a surprise," she said. "I guess I am more emotionally sensitive than I let on. I need to better express this somehow." You may uncover a similar response when you see your results, or you may get exactly the breakdown you expected. Stay open to learning more about yourself.

This assessment is here to help you get started on your journey toward *Mamaste*. It's meant to serve you and give you the tools to grow and get the most out of motherhood. And it's not a definitive test, either. Your primary expression can also change over time or in response to a particular situation, so always feel free to go back and redo the assessment if you feel you need a refresher.

MAMA TYPE QUIZ

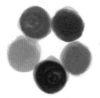

How to do it: Please read through the following paired statements and choose the one that is the truest for you. If the statements don't resonate perfectly for you, please choose the one that feels close enough, or that happens most of the time. It's good to be relaxed and in the moment when taking the assessment, and try not to overthink it!

1.

After you have a disagreement with someone, you don't hold a grudge. **D**

People ask you for things because they know you will always do it. **B**

2.

Everybody wants you on the planning committee for their fundraiser because you know how to get shit done. **A**

When it comes to raising your children, the more people to help guide you, the merrier. **C**

3.

When trying to make decisions, you look to outside sources to seek your answers rather than looking within. **C**

It's hard for people to get to know the real you because you guard your feelings carefully. **D**

4.

Your family vacations are planned with an hour-by-hour itinerary. **A**

Reality is overrated. **D**

5.

Being creative is how you express yourself. **E**

You tend to sweep your emotions under the carpet instead of dealing with them. **D**

6.

Your own needs are usually at the bottom of your to-do list. **B**

Making mistakes makes you cringe. **A**

7.

You have a unique perspective. **E**

Like a chameleon, you can fit in just about anywhere. **B**

8.

Because you're so capable, people expect a lot from you. **A**

People often come to you for your ability to see the big picture with a thousand-foot view. **E**

9.

If an opportunity to join a mom's group or take a parenting class comes your way, you are the first to sign up. **C**

You let things go easily in order to avoid conflict. **B**

10.

Your to-do lists guide your life. **A**

You don't often worry about the outcome of the situation. **D**

11.

Following the rules makes you cringe. **E**

You're happy to play a supportive role to an established leader. **B**

12.

You are a master of multitasking. **A**

You do you and live your own way without caring about what others think. **E**

13.

You know who you are and are not a pushover. **E**

You tend to think your way through life instead of feeling it out. **A**

14.

You roll your eyes and want to punch someone when another mom tells you how you should parent your child. **E**

When you're socializing with fellow moms, you love to pick their brains about parenting techniques and how they're handling motherhood. **C**

15.

Within a week of getting a positive pregnancy test, you hired an entire birthing team and researched everything about pregnancy, birth, and parenting choices. **A**

You let your doctor guide your pregnancy choices and were happy to take advice from friends and family along the way. **B**

16.

If a person of authority tells you to do something, your instinct is to do the opposite. **E**

When it comes to big decisions, you will poll any- and everyone you possibly can to get their opinion. **C**

17.

You often find yourself lying in bed at night worrying about what might happen in the future. **C**

You don't allow yourself to get hurt emotionally very often. **D**

18.

Other moms might view you as a lone wolf. **E**

You ask for and accept help easily. **C**

19.

You prefer to be liberated from the complications of life. **D**

Organizing is your favorite hobby. **A**

20.

It's hard to get you to change your opinion. **E**

You transition with ease and adjust to what's happening around you. **B**

21.

There is nothing like a little competition to ignite the fire in you to win. **A**

If you are having a hard time getting it all done, you don't hesitate to ask for help. **C**

22.

When you believe in something, you are not easily swayed by other opinions. **E**

When shit gets too real, you'd prefer not to deal. **D**

23.

In a perfect world, someone else would take on all of your responsibility for you. **C**

When it comes to favors or requests, you often say yes when you really mean no. **B**

24.

When out with friends, you'd prefer to talk about the latest fashion trends than the state of the world. **D**

You'd rather have a root canal than get into a confrontation. **B**

25.

If there is an issue at your child's school, you are not afraid to lead the fight to right the wrong that is happening. **E**

You tend to keep things light and on the surface when communicating with people. **D**

26.

You often use "Dr. Google," and the information you find causes you to panic with uncontrollable fear. **C**

Drama is for the movies, not your life. **B**

27.

Your own instincts don't seem reliable enough; you would rather trust someone else's advice. **C**

You prefer to do things by yourself because no one will handle it as well as you can. **A**

28.

You have a childlike sense of wonder. **C**

You have a hard time staying present in the moment. **D**

29.

You disconnect from your body and numb out (overeating, over-drinking, overworking, etc.) to avoid feeling pain. **D**

You often feel depleted because you can't say no; you're con-stantly doing things for others and overextending yourself. **B**

30.

You tend to get agitated when things don't go as planned. **A**

It's great to be included in others' plans because all the details are already managed, so you can enjoy the ride. **B**

Now tally up the number of letters, and fill them in here:

A: **B:**   **C:**   **D:**   **E:**

Remember, the highest score indicates your primary mama expression, but you'll also score in the other expressions, even if it's very low. It is possible to have two or three expressions tie as the highest score, which means you are well balanced between these expressions. You'll read much more about all five expressions in the following chapters, but here's a brief overview of each:

(A) Action: Action Mamas are excellent planners, incredible leaders, and know how to get shit done. They are take-charge women, but they're also prone to planning and solving things *too* much, leaving little space for anything else to unfold.

(B) Flow: Flow Mamas may seem effortlessly easy-breezy and able to adapt to anything without frustration. But all this "going with the flow" often comes at the expense of the Flow Mama herself. She can have a hard time expressing needs and preferences when she does have them, and sometimes she allows herself to be talked into things that aren't comfortable, simply to avoid confrontation.

(C) Vulnerable: The Vulnerable Mama harnesses her natural curiosity and openness, seeks out extra attention and support, and wisely uses "the village" to help her raise her family. But without grounding forces, the Vulnerable Mama can spiral into her own anxieties and fears, and start spinning out of control.

(D) Free: The Free Mama isn't super attached to outcomes, which lets her approach tasks and opportunities without worrying about the future. She may have unresolved trauma, and often her strategy for dealing with difficulties is to plow right through, doing whatever she needs to make it through the day.

(E) Rebel: Strong, forward-thinking, and often blazing her own unique path, the Rebel Mama beats to her own drum and does things on her terms—standing up for what she believes in even if she stands alone. While the Rebel Mama is already able to confidently express her authenticity, she can struggle with feeling rushed or pushed to make a decision before she's ready to get there.

Are you surprised by the results or are they pretty much what you assumed? This is an attitudinal assessment, not a personality assessment, which means that the results can change over time, especially when you deepen your consciousness and make shifts in your focus and behavior. Once you see where you are, you can start to use this book as your guide. You may also notice where to pull up and integrate more of one expression or back off and soften another.

The beauty of living in *Mamaste* is that we are all one. *The mother in me is the mother in you.* Take a deep cleansing breath as you step forward into a world of greater balance, wholeness, and harmony.

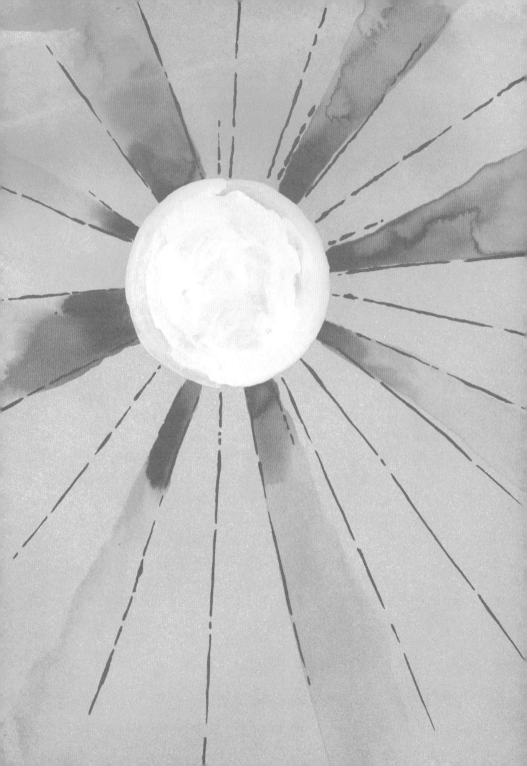

chapter three

ACTION MAMA

Just Wanna Get Things Done

~~~~~~~~~~~~~~~~~~~~

Dear Action Mama: I know your time is valuable, so I'm going to get right to the point. We all know you are an excellent planner and an incredible leader, and you know how to get shit done. I'd hire you to run my business in a second! You always have a plan, and your friends and family are so grateful (even if they don't always show it) for your amazing energy and problem-solving skills. You're a take-charge, kick-ass kind of woman.

But the strange thing about parenting, as you've probably discovered, is that it's full of surprises. And if you're prone to planning and solving and controlling things *too* much, it leaves little space for anything else to unfold. I'll give you an example: I often tell clients who are trying to get pregnant that overplanning kills the magic in the bedroom. Any of you who have *scheduled* baby-making know exactly what I mean! But this principle extends to a lot of other areas in life as well. By connecting with the other expressions of Flow, Vulnerability, Rebelliousness, and Freedom—and you have them, even if you don't think you do—you'll become more flexible, worry less about the outcome, and enjoy the moment a lot more.

Do you ever feel agitated and upset when things don't go according to plan? What would happen if you allowed life to unfold a bit more organically, without managing every aspect of it? Usually, when I ask my Action Mama clients these questions, they admit they're scared to relax, because if they're not holding it all together, everything—including them—will fall apart. This anxiety and distrust is what often drives the need to control in the first place. You may be thinking, *I can't relax! That's just not me!* and I hear you. I would never ask you to be something you're not. This book is all about staying true to yourself and deepening your self-awareness. So instead of trying to turn *off* your primary expression of Action, what if you dialed up more of the other expressions to help find harmony and balance within yourself?

Being an Action Mama is all about finding strength, structure, and authority to feel more centered and in charge. As an Action Mama, you tend to channel your energy into gathering information, focusing on goals, and stepping into leadership roles in order to build a solid foundation and framework for your family. You're usually extremely capable of juggling multiple priorities, keeping a well-organized home, and planning ahead in both your personal and professional lives. You know these attributes help you get things done more efficiently! If you find satisfaction in making lists, preparing in advance, and balancing busy schedules, your primary expression may be Action.

The challenge for this expression is not to let all the planning trap you into a system that's too rigid—this is where you can benefit greatly from tapping into expressions like Flow and Free. Action Mamas often hold themselves to an impossibly high standard, and use their meticulous and polished nature to conceal feelings of anxiety and guilt. Because you're so capable, people expect a lot from you, and that can make it difficult to seek and receive much-needed help when you really need it.

✳ EMBRACE LESS CONTROL

Many of the Action Mamas I've worked with have flourished by establishing structure and systems within their daily routines— as long as it includes room for flexibility and fluidity when things don't go as planned (and as you probably know, they often don't!). Sarah created a strict sleep schedule for her kids every night. Without fail, by 7 p.m., they were in their pj's, and by 7:30, they were in bed. Even though it meant they often missed out on neighborhood get-togethers or family events, Sarah felt this kind of structure was good for her kids. One Saturday night at a friend's house, she found herself having a meaningful conversation with a new mom friend, and their kids were having a blast in the playroom. Suddenly, she tensed up. It was 6:50—*Shit, we have to go.* When she explained the situation, her new friend said, "I wish you could stay a bit longer. What's the worst thing that would happen if the kids miss their bedtime routine?"

Sarah thought, *Well, they might be a little tired and cranky the next day, but it would be so nice to be able to hang out for another hour or two since everyone's getting along so well.* After that evening, she started to reconsider some of her other strict parenting rules, too. By loosening the rope just a little, she allowed herself the space to live in the moment and keep her life from feeling too restrictive.

Imagine a beautiful tree that bends and sways with the breeze. Now imagine a tree that's rigid and stiff, unable to move as much. If the wind is too strong, a branch will eventually snap off and fall to the ground. When life gets chaotic, it's tempting to try to exert even *more* control, but like the tree in a storm, this is when you need flexibility the most. It requires you to trust that you'll be able to weather the storm—and I know that's not an easy leap of faith. But in order to find balance, you have to soften your energy and trust that the universe has your back—meaning, give yourself room for unexpected possibilities, mistakes, twists, and turns. Often it's in these moments when we learn the most about ourselves and can grow.

*PLAN WHAT YOU CAN

Brooke's goal was to breastfeed for at least six months, and she had invested in a hospital-grade pump, nursing bras, and a bottle system for daycare when she returned to work. She'd seen other working moms pump successfully for up to a year and felt she should be able to accomplish the same thing for her baby. For months she struggled daily—dragging the pump back and forth on her commute, and nursing throughout the night—until she felt completely overwhelmed and exhausted. The idea of breastfeeding was driving her crazy, and the only thing keeping her going was a deep sense of guilt that she couldn't "keep up" with other working moms.

After a few excruciatingly long pumping sessions that yielded only a few ounces of milk, she broke down and decided she needed a plan B: to find the best organic formula to add as a substitute to her dwindling milk supply. By allowing herself to reevaluate her original goals and find a new goal that fit her lifestyle and supported her baby better, Brooke let go of the one thing that wasn't working and quickly began to enjoy all the other things that came more easily as a new mom.

how to get to plan b

First, how do you know when your original plan isn't working? You're likely feeling overwhelmed, stressed, or perhaps angry and lashing out at the wrong person or situation.

> Get out of the tornado—sit down and take a few deep breaths. Pausing to stop and think is a huge step itself, and will allow you to gather your thoughts before you can redirect your energy.

> Make a list of what you can change and what you can't. This will help you focus on what's possible.

> Talk to someone who is not judgmental. When you're in a vulnerable situation, you don't need anyone making you feel guilty or second-guess your instincts.

> Create a new plan—plan B—that allows for additional tweaks and changes. Chances are, you'll need more flexibility down the road, and by leaving space to maneuver, you won't feel as stuck as you did the first time around.

✳ THE BENEFITS OF ACTION FOR OTHER EXPRESSIONS

The benefits of Action Mama may seem obvious for the other expressions—who doesn't want to be more organized?—but it's not always that easy to tap into an alpha style. Rebel Mamas may feel stifled at first by a set schedule, but if it leaves plenty of room to be spontaneous, it can help them create consistency and common ground. Similarly, Vulnerable Mamas may feel intimidated by the idea of taking on a leadership role, but if practiced slowly and with support, they can build confidence and a sense of ownership within their families and communities. Adopting the elements of Action Mama to fit your own personality will help you grow in your primary expression and also honor and respect those seemingly "effortless" moms who may be struggling just as much as anyone else underneath.

If you're not primarily an Action Mama but have a friend who embodies this expression, why not reap the benefits of her natural talents? Treat your well-organized BFF to a coffee or lunch and pick her brain about the research she's done on something you need, or get her ideas on organizing your kids' schedule or playroom—you'll be surprised at how excited she is to share her hard-earned knowledge, and you'll walk away all the wiser.

✳ RELATING TO THE ACTION MAMA

Carrie can never keep dates straight and is chronically late to playdates and school events. After a hectic week of running around and feeling completely out of control, she bumped into her friend Jane, who always seemed so put-together. Taking a chance, Carrie opened up about her lack of organization, and to her surprise, Jane offered to invite her to important school events using a shared Google calendar with reminders. It was a win-win solution—Jane felt flattered to be useful, and Carrie was grateful for a little help with her busy schedule.

Honoring an Action Mama can be as simple as acknowledging her efforts, whether she plans incredible birthday parties or never misses a planning meeting. It may appear easy for her, but she's working hard, and chances are your praise will go a long way toward making her feel valued and appreciated.

But what if you run into an overzealous Action Mama? There's no doubt you've seen one taking the lead in your mom's group and directing everyone—her take-charge approach can make you feel as though you can't get a word in! But before you roll your eyes and take another swig of your wine, remember—she's doing her best the way she knows how. Empathy is key, no matter what expression you're dealing with. What would it look like if you stepped into her scuffless shoes? Try asking her if she'd be willing to head up a committee nobody else can handle—you really need her amazing organizational talents and energy. Chances are, she'll step up to the task and feel useful, and you'll be relieved when her great energy is focused on a specific project instead of on micro-managing everything.

✳ THE PROBLEM WITH PERFECTION

It's okay to mess up. Perfectionism is dangerous and doesn't allow us to take risks, because we live in fear of failure all the time.

—DR. CARLI SOLOMON SNYDER

It's hard not to feel pressure to be a "perfect mom" these days, with images of the ideal modern mom coming at you from all angles. *I don't know how she does it!* is the common refrain, and there's a pervasive idea that being too busy is a sign of success.

Action Mamas actually struggle more with this ideal than others. Because they are so capable, they feel they *should* measure up to a high standard. I spoke to psychologist Dr. Stephanie Askari about the myth of the perfect mom, and she gave me some insight into her own story:

> At some point, it became compellingly and unavoidably clear to me that I didn't want my daughter to become a perfectionist like me. I could tell her until I was blue in the face to just try her best, but if I didn't walk the walk myself, she, too, would fall victim to the vice of perfectionism. Loving my daughter more than my own need to be perfect is what helped me let things go.
>
> I don't think perfect moms raise better kids. I think good-enough moms raise healthier kids—kids who are resilient, compassionate toward themselves and others, and willing to make mistakes and learn from them. Good-enough moms make mistakes themselves and are willing to own up to that and make things right when they can; that process teaches kids invaluable lessons.

One of my clients, Amy, told me she couldn't stop shopping for her soon-to-be baby. She wanted everything to be perfect, but she felt completely lost. She compulsively bought three cribs, four bouncers, and multiple Pack 'n Plays, and put them all over her home. Crying, she said, "Lori, I can't stop! I need help." I asked her to draw a picture of her ideal self—the woman and mom she thought she was supposed to be—and we named her Ginger. Ginger had a supermodel body with big perky boobs, long legs, and flowing hair, holding a perfect baby—and just the ridiculousness of it made us both laugh out loud. By naming her alter ego and examining this unrealistic expectation for herself, Amy was able to shift her awareness and shed light on the truth behind her feelings. She now understands the triggers when Ginger shows up and has the awareness to tell her, "You're not real, so take a hike!"

✳ LET IT GOOOOO

Take some time to relax, take your bra off, and chill the f*ck out. You've earned it! This is especially true for Action Mamas, who often see motherhood as an opportunity to get even *more* things done. Let me let you in on a little secret, ladies. By taking time for yourself to relax, YOU ARE *ACTUALLY* DOING SOMETHING. Recharging your batteries will allow you to be more efficient, energized, and focused.

I know, I know. You can't just relax. It's not in your

nature. In order to let go, you need to check a few things off your list and *then* you can surrender.

A client of mine was in labor, and before heading to the hospital, we stopped by her doctor's office to have her checked so as not to arrive too early. Her intention was to have an unmedicated birth. She was already six centimeters dilated, so I encouraged her to walk it out and use gravity to help the baby along. The hospital was only two miles away, so we set out. As we walked, she kept texting her mom and husband to-do lists, and she asked her husband to pull over so she could make sure the hospital bags were packed properly in the car. Once she knew everything was in order, including calling the pediatrician and the placenta person to give them a heads-up, she was then able to surrender and let go. We kept walking right to the hospital, and she pushed her baby out. Let's just say we all got our steps in that day.

I'm here to give you full permission to be lazy. Seriously. It's freeing to detach from responsibilities, and dropping into a decompressed state is important for your well-being. Whether you prefer binge-watching TV, curling up with a good book, or scrolling through Instagram (say hi to me @lbreggy!), it's okay to use downtime as self-care. Action Mamas in particular need to let themselves feel worthy of "free time" instead of trying to pack a million things into every second.

ask for help when you need it

Action Mamas tend to be doers—driven to be efficient and goal-oriented and prioritizing to-do's over all else. This tends to be more of a masculine energy. It's hard to *feel* anything when you're so laser-focused on getting things done. Your independent nature means you don't like relying on others; you'd prefer to be in control, and that protects you from disappointment, hurt, or regret. Your nonstop pace leaves little room to receive help from others. Accessing an expression of Vulnerability can help you soften, get more comfortable with your feelings, and connect more deeply to yourself and your family.

Even the most intimate relationships can be difficult for Action Mamas to navigate. Lucy's one-year-old daughter caught a stomach flu at daycare, so she stayed home with her. By the second day, Lucy was sick, too. She thought about asking her husband to come home early to help out but hesitated—*I should be able to handle this, right? And besides, he's busy.* By the time her husband arrived home late that evening, Lucy was completely on edge and exhausted—and he felt terrible not knowing how bad things were.

It's important to remember that nobody is a mind reader, so if you need someone to step up for you, you gotta ask for it! True intimacy in any relationship or friendship can occur only when you allow yourself to be vulnerable—vulnerability is not a weakness, it's often a sign of great strength.

Action Mamas can benefit from developing friendships with Vulnerable Mamas because they already live in a realm of asking and receiving. Vulnerable Mamas understand this need and don't see it as a weakness.

integrate rebel energy

To practice getting out of your set routine and integrating some Rebel energy, take yourself on an adventure without needing a plane ticket. Simply take a different route or try a new thing: change up your drive to work, choose a new coffee spot, start at the opposite end of the grocery store. It can be that simple, and it really works to break up the need for constant structure and sameness. Once you get comfortable, maybe once a month try something really new, such as taking your kids on a nature hike (if that's not usually your thing), or cranking up the music on a Friday night and getting your whole family to sing along to favorite songs. It may sound counterintuitive, but you can practice spontaneity!

You may never be the mom waltzing into Back-to-School Night in a flowy caftan, offering to host a séance as a fundraiser—but you *can* access a deeper well of creativity and magic. The key is to practice allowing the process to unfold and savoring each step instead of pushing toward the finished product. Whether you're finger painting with your kids or looking for new ways to make family vacations feel more exciting, you can benefit greatly by giving yourself permission to *play* and letting your intuition lead the way.

Maria's weekends were always jam-packed with activities, from birthday parties to dance lessons and family functions. After a particularly exhausting Saturday she felt overwhelmed. *Forget it*, she thought, *nobody's enjoying this*. She canceled all Sunday plans and let the family sleep late. They cooked breakfast in their pajamas, played board games, grabbed BBQ supplies at a local market, and that night, they all snuggled up together to watch a favorite movie. It was the best day Maria could remember in a long time, and it changed her whole family's perspective on spending time together.

Action Mamas are amazingly capable, talented, multifaceted mothers and women. You do a lot, and it's important to let yourself feel appreciated, supported, and loved, regardless of whether or not you've checked off everything on your to-do list. Practicing self-love may feel silly or unnecessary, but I don't mean treating yourself to a mani-pedi (although having someone rub your feet is always a worthwhile luxury!). What I mean is actually trusting the universe to have your back—by asking for help when you need it, letting others occasionally lead the way, and letting go when things feel too forced or frustrating. Finding a balance of control and release can unlock a life of joy and fulfillment that may not ever come from the pursuit of "having it all."

*MANIFESTING MAGIC

You're ultra-organized, prepared, and sensibly dressed—even your kids look as if they walked out of the pages of a J.Crew catalog. This is how you show the world you take pride in yourself. But what if your perfectionist nature is holding you hostage? A lot of Action Mamas wish they could be more creative and impulsive, but their need for order and control makes it difficult to let go and connect with their more free-spirited sides. Rebel Mamas do this naturally—they tend to be artists, dreamers, and visionaries, and they march to the beat of their own drum without even realizing it. They're not competing or comparing themselves to anyone else because they are authentic and doing their own thing in their own time. To an Action Mama, this sounds damn near impossible! But it's not—you just need to tap into your Rebel expression.

action mama toolkit

✳ Action Recipe:
Lemon Rose Hips Tonic

When you can't seem to do it right, and you don't feel that you're enough, trace minerals and adaptogenic herbs can help calm the adrenals and soothe the heart. Lemon and rose hips (which you can find at health food stores or online) come together in a bright, refreshing tonic crafted by Heng Ou that can be sipped any time of the day or night.

SERVES 4

- *1 tablespoon dried rose hips*
- *1-inch (2.5-cm) knob of fresh ginger, peeled*
- *2 tablespoons fresh lemon juice*
- *1 tablespoon honey*

➤ Bring 4 cups (960 ml) water to a boil in a small pot, along with the dried rose hips and fresh ginger. Turn the heat down to low and simmer for 20 minutes, covered.

➤ Turn off the heat, add the fresh lemon juice, and let it all steep for 5 minutes. Strain and sweeten with honey (as desired) and sip throughout the day.

✳ Action Supplements:
Maintain a Healthy Balance

Elissa Goodman recommends these nutritional supplements to calm your nervous system and balance your body where it needs it most.

Gaia Holy Basil: Basil helps to maintain balance and calmness, allowing more room for making things happen without controlling them.

Gaia Valerian Root: This root helps you stay calm and present so you don't feel the need to manage everything all the time.

Calm Magnesium Powder: This supplement can also help you feel calm and provides helpful nutrients to relax your organs, muscles, and digestive system.

✳ Action Oils:
Calm Down and Find Your Focus

All these oils can be diffused, added to a bath, or worn as a healing perfume. A lot of essential oil blends often contain hidden chemicals, so I recommend Young Living Essential Oils for their high-grade quality and purity.

YOUNG LIVING ESSENTIAL OILS

Stress Away Blend: to wash tension away

Peace & Calming Blend: to relax the body and mind

Vetiver Oil: to calm and focus the mind

✳ Action Crystals:
Reflect with Clarity

When you first get your crystal, you have to solidify your bond. As with with any relationship, it takes time for your energies to sync. For a crystal to purify your energy, you have to first return the gesture and cleanse its energy. You can let your crystal bathe outside in the light of the sun or moon for at least four hours, or place it on the soil or hang it on the branch of a healthy house-plant for twenty-four hours. Then sit quietly, holding the stone in both your hands. Visualize your intention for the crystals. The stone is listening. Giving your crystal a job allows you to set your intention for the work you'll do together. It's okay to get specific! After programming the crystal with your intention, your crystal is now activated. Heather Askinosie has chosen these crystals specifically to help Action Mamas find balance.

Clear Quartz: This stone allows Action Mamas to solve their issues by doing what they do best—plan! When an Action Mama finds herself becoming overly controlling or ignoring one aspect of her life to concentrate too intently on another, she can use clear quartz to program the intention of release and clarity. The clarity that clear quartz lends will assist her in recognizing the perspectives of others, as well as show her how she can remain passionate and devoted to every area of her life through achiev-ing the right balance.

Snowflake Obsidian: When the stress of all that the Action Mama feels she needs to plan and control builds up, she can use snowflake obsidian to break through the pattern of self-imposed anxiety. Snowflake obsidian will remind the Action Mama that life is not black and white, success or failure. There can be successes in faults, and faults in successes, and snowflake obsidian's mirror-like quality allows Action Mama to reflect on each of these subtle nuances.

Red Jasper: This stone empowers Action Mamas to tap into their greatest strengths, so they can strive to take action, move forward, and be fearless in every challenge that presents itself.

action yoga:
get out of your head and into your heart

Action Mamas tend to spend a lot of time in their heads (thinking, assessing, worrying) and often need a little help bringing energy toward their hearts (feeling, intuiting). Too much action can mean you don't have the time to drop in on yourself and acknowledge what you might need or how you feel. This yoga practice will also help connect you with love, gratitude, forgiveness, and compassion for yourself and for others. It softens your energy and opens your heart to remind you how amazing you are and how abundant your life truly is!

You can do this as an entire sequence or pick and choose individual poses as they fit with your current mood or energy level.

Suggested props: *2 yoga blocks, 1 yoga strap, 2 to 3 blankets, rose oil (optional)*

- Start off in a comfortable seated position, and if you choose, rub 3 drops of rose oil on your heart. Rose oil is the healing oil for the heart chakra. It connects you with feminine energy and helps connect you to love and compassion for yourself and others.

- Next, close your eyes, then take the pointer and middle finger of your right hand and tap your heart gently for 1 minute. This will help move some energy and wake up the heart area. As you are tapping, set your intention for your practice to open and soften your heart, to let go of anything that might be blocking you from giving or receiving love, or connecting more deeply with feelings of gratitude, compassion, forgiveness, and joy.

✳ Hands at the Wall

- Stand and place your hands flat on a wall, shoulder distance apart, feet hip-width apart. Walk your feet back until your arms are straight and parallel to each other. Take a slow deep breath into the back of your heart, and as you exhale, allow your chest to sink down toward the floor. Often we get carried away and fixated on all that we *haven't* accomplished— now, think of a few things you have done lately that you are really proud of. Take a second to acknowledge and take this in by breathing it in deeply. As you exhale, soften and relax your chest, dropping it even deeper to the ground. Repeat a total of 5 times.

✳ Doorway Heart Opener

- Standing in a doorway, place your elbows, forearms, and palms flat on each side of the door frame. Step your right foot forward and press your chest through your arms. Inhale deeply into your chest and lungs and exhale, allowing your chest and shoulders to relax. Take 3 to 5 slow deep breaths, each one filled with something you were grateful for today.

✳ Arm Circles

- Standing, stretch your arms out to either side, parallel to the floor, and begin to circle your arms, moving from small circles to larger circles for 30 seconds; then reverse direction for 30 seconds.

✳ Windmill

- With your arms still stretched out to the sides, make fists with your hands. Turn your body slightly to the right, swinging your arms loosely so that your fists aim to gently tap your heart and the back of your chest at the same time. Repeat about 30 times (or 1 minute).

✳ Shake Out

- Still standing, imagine you are shaking out any energy you may be holding in your heart that isn't serving you—stress, disappointment, judgment, anger, jealousy, sadness. Now shake your arms and legs out as if you are freeing them of these feelings. Shake them fast and hard—be free of it! Let that shit go! You can even say it out loud: "I let go of the anger I felt after what my mother-in-law said last night!"

✳ Shoulder Opener

- Grab a strap in both hands, holding it in front of you, down by your hips, with arms straight a little bit more than shoulder distance apart (if your shoulders are tight, you might need to open your arms more). Inhale, lift the strap up to the top of your head, and exhale, letting the strap fall behind you. Now inhale and lift the strap up behind you, and exhale as you bring it down in front of you. Repeat this for 10 rounds, thinking or chanting "I am love" on each inhale, and on the exhale, "Love I am." Exhale and inhale.

✳ Alternating Chest Opener

- Still holding on to the strap from Shoulder Opener, lift your right hand over your head and bend your elbow slightly behind you. Position your left arm behind your lower back and grab on to the other end of the strap. Slowly crawl your hands closer together. If your shoulders and chest are loose, you can skip the strap and try to clasp your hands together. Take a deep breath into your chest, and, as you exhale, fold your body forward. Hold and breathe in and out a few times, then switch sides.

✳ Love Gun

- Standing with feet hip-width apart, clasp your hands behind your back (if your shoulders are tight, you can use a strap). Inhale, and lift your chest up. Think of five people you feel super grateful to have in your life. As you inhale, think about why they're such a blessing to you, and exhale out your love and gratitude for them.

✳ Child's Pose Stretch

- Return to a seated position with your legs and ankles tucked underneath you. Lower your torso forward so your arms are stretched out along the floor in front of you. Walk your hands to the left, take a deep breath, and acknowledge three things that make you a great mom. Exhale and relax. Now walk your hands to the right, take a deep breath, and acknowledge three things that make you feel proud of your child(ren). Exhale and relax. Walk your hands back to the center, breathe in and out a few more times, and soften the rib cage to relax.

☀ Love Thyself Meditation

- Sit cross-legged in front of a mirror (if you don't have one that reaches the floor, it's fine to position a smaller mirror in front of you). If you have one, hold a rose quartz with both hands on your chest where your heart is. Begin to move your hands clockwise in a circular movement. With your hands moving on your heart, stare into your own eyes in the mirror. If distracting thoughts arise, bring the focus back to your reflection; if negative thoughts arise, think about something positive about yourself. For example: *I look old*—I look wise. *I hate my arms*—I wore my baby everywhere.

- Sit in this meditation for 1 to 3 minutes, continuing to change your focus back to the positive. The longer you can do this, the more powerful and healing the work will be!

- Next, bring your hands into a prayer position, and thank yourself for making this effort and for your miraculous life. Too often we take the simplest things for granted, and it is always a worthwhile reminder to acknowledge the food on your table, the fresh air that you breathe, the fresh water you drink, and the roof over your head. From deep within your heart, send love and prayers to those throughout the world who may live without.

- Finally, if there is someone in your own immediate life who needs extra love or positive energy (including yourself), offer them your final thoughts. *Mamaste.*

action affirmations:
trust yourself

I like to tape affirmations to my mirror so I see them every morning—it's a great way to start the day off right. Take a look at the list below and circle at least three that really jump out at you. Type or write them out and put them in a place you'll be sure to see every day. You could even type them into your phone as your alarm reminder text!

Now here's the fun part: Actually say each affirmation three times, out loud. Don't be afraid to sound silly or weird (practice in the bathroom or anywhere you can be truly alone!). By chanting the affirmations out loud, you'll implant them in your subconscious, and eventually they will become a part of your conscious reality.

I TRUST THE FLOW OF LIFE.

IT'S SAFE FOR ME TO SLOW DOWN.

THERE IS NO SUCH THING AS PERFECT.

I SURRENDER.

NOBODY HAS IT ALL FIGURED OUT.

I SOFTEN.

I LEAVE ROOM FOR MAGIC.

I ALLOW AND DESERVE MORE TIME FOR PLAY.

I TRUST DIVINE TIMING.

PATIENCE IS A VIRTUE.

MY LIFE WON'T FALL APART
IF I LET GO OF SOME CONTROL.

I ENJOY THE PROCESS ONE STEP AT A TIME.

I AM ENOUGH.

action meditation:
breathe and balance

As an Action Mama, you do a lot. When you give 100 percent it's more like 500 percent. You're diligent with a laser-sharp focus that helps you accomplish what many can't even imagine! You're uniquely capable of checking off a long to-do list and staying on top of what your kids and family need. But what about yourself? Sometimes taking a break from all this "doing" can actually help you recharge so that you're able to get back to the task at hand more energetically. Simply taking the time to wander—even in your own mind—can help you find balance.

This is a worthwhile break to connect with yourself and find balance mentally and emotionally, written by Michele Meiche. Take 20 minutes for yourself. You deserve it; and this will actually make you even more efficient in the long run.

As you read these words, let your breathing slow down and start to become more present in the moment. You're going to give yourself the time to go on a journey of your inner land-scape that will help center your mind and body and refresh your spirit.

Breathe in for a count of 3, pause for a count of 3, and breathe out slowly for a count of 3.

Breathe in for a count of 3, pause for a count of 3, and breathe out slowly for a count of 3.

Breathe in for a count of 3 even slower than before, pause for a count of 3, and breathe out slowly for a count of 3.

Now, begin breathing in for a count of 1, pause for a count of 1, and breathe out for a count of 1.

Let your breath return to its own natural rhythm. Notice how much slower your breathing is and how much calmer you feel. Now imagine yourself walking on a trail. This trail can be an actual trail you have walked before, or it can be one that now appears in your mind. Perhaps it's a composite of trails you've visited before. There is something familiar about this trail and so you feel safe, peaceful, and calm. As you walk along the trail, you begin to look around and take in all the sights and sounds.

You look around and see the plants, flowers, and trees. Walk slowly as you take in all the nature. You are becoming more present to the natural world around you.

As you walk farther up the trail, you begin to hear the sounds of water. Perhaps you can feel the air that is crisp, yet warm. It is the perfect temperature and the perfect time for you. Walk up a little farther, and you will see a part in the trail that begins to curve to the right. Let yourself walk slowly on this part of the trail. You begin to notice something new. There is a lightness in your step and a sense of ease as you turn the corner.

To the right of the trail is a large tree with cascading branches that offer wonderful shade. As you walk toward the tree, you notice to the left of the tree is a peaceful flowing river. You walk over to the tree and sit down to watch the river flow. Along the bank of the river are the most beautiful flowers and foliage. There is such a peace and calm here. It the perfect place for you to sit and watch the river flow and take a rest. Sit down at the base of the tree shaded by the leaves with arching branches overhead and lean back against the trunk, feeling it support you.

As you watch the river flow, you notice a leaf from the tree floating in the river. Watch how the leaf is embraced and carried by the water.

This landscape is so calm and serene that you stay here for a while taking in all the peaceful energy and the calm of the river, watching the gentle flow of nature.

Take your time at this special place.

When you are ready, come back to your everyday focus.

Take 3 deep breaths with a slow inhale and exhale and say in your own mind:

Just for today . . .

Just for this moment . . .

I will let it all be.

I let go and accept what is right now in front of me . . .

Breathe in . . . *I am perfect as I am and trusting all that is in the flow for me.*

Breathe out . . . *I am allowing all to be . . .*

deepening your self-awareness

Answer these questions in order as they build upon each other, to continue understanding and connecting with your inner Action Mama expression:

1. Where does or where has your Action expression shown up in your life?

2. What do you resist or find the most off-putting about Action Mamas?

3. Where do you resist this aspect of the Action Mama within yourself?

4. Who's your favorite Action Mama, and what do you admire about her?

5. Where can you see parts of her reflected in you?

6. How might your life change from integrating more of your Action expression into your life and being?

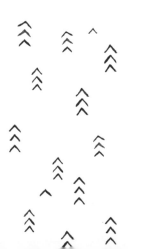

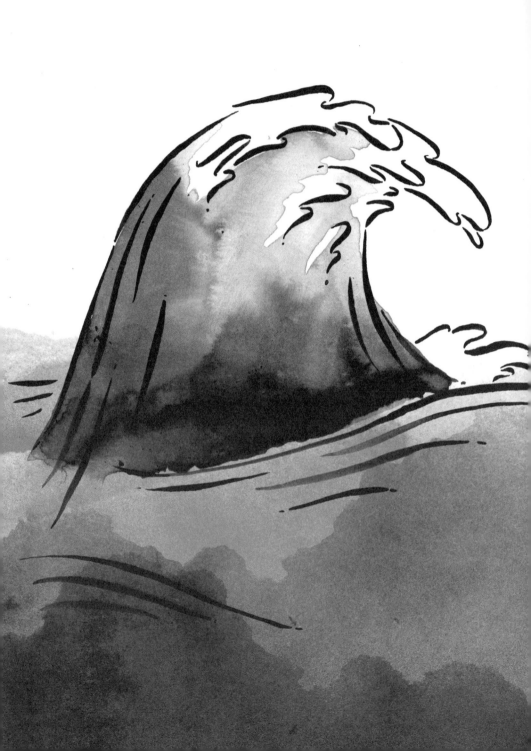

chapter four

FLOW MAMA

Easy Like Sunday Morning

~~~~~~~~~~~~~~~~~~~~~

Easy, breezy, beautiful . . . That's you, Flow Mama.
A loyal friend and the perfect wing woman, you're a dream come
true for anyone lucky enough to know you. When you're around,
there's rarely conflict, as you're naturally open to suggestions
and able to adapt effortlessly, as drama-free is your happy place.
Your easygoing nature and ability to switch gears without friction
means you don't need to impose strict rules for yourself or your
family. And when the shit hits the fan and everyone else freaks
out, you're already adjusting to the new direction and cooperating
with others. Why contribute to the chaos when you can flow right
into the new plan? You make life feel easy and fun for everyone
around you, which in turn brings you and all those around you a
sense of satisfaction and happiness.

But (and you knew there'd be a *but*, right?) all of this "going with the flow" often comes at your own expense. You may be genuinely happy going along with the group 99 percent of the time, but what happens when you do have a difference of opinion? Part of your desire to say yes is your gift of flexibility, but part of it is also your anxiety around saying no. (By the way, this issue isn't unique just to Flow Mamas—many of us tend to struggle with saying no!) Because you don't like to rock the boat, you can have a hard time expressing your own needs and preferences when you do have them. And others may not hear you right away, or they may be surprised when you take a stand. God forbid you should actually set a boundary. Because of your aversion to the word *no*, you may often find yourself taking on more than you can handle, which leaves you feeling overwhelmed, depleted, and resentful. Put simply, you can easily be taken advantage of, and that's no way to *Mamaste*.

Many of the Flow Mamas I've worked with say that motherhood adds a whole new dimension to this struggle. Being natural people pleasers, Flow Mamas have a hard time setting boundaries and often put their own needs last on their list of priorities. This may work in the short term, but you may find that being the easy, breezy, happy-go-lucky girl starts to feel less important than standing strong in your own convictions, both for yourself and for your family. When it was just you, this might have worked out, but now that you are responsible for others (your children, partner, and even pets), being too loosey-goosey in your approach might actually backfire. Motherhood usually comes with a few extra moving parts all at once, and without structure, boundaries, or even a preliminary plan, things will quickly start to feel out of control.

✳ FIND YOUR VOICE IN THE FLOW

The good news is that you possess four other expressions to tap into in order to find the strength to thrive. Setting boundaries and standing strong is something Rebel Mamas do so well. Don't let the word *rebel* intimidate you! Rebel Mamas tend to fly under the radar and aren't usually competitive with others. Their real strength comes from an inner sense of personal truth and confidence; they're not afraid to let someone down or upset someone if it means sticking to their core beliefs. This steely core is what you'll work on developing in order to practice saying no without guilt or fear.

Jill was a classic people pleaser—she said yes to favors that often inconvenienced her and found it especially difficult to refuse her neighbors, whom she saw on a daily basis. She and her husband had originally fallen in love with their tight-knit suburban community, but Jill was starting to feel like the actual doormat on her front steps. Last-minute request to watch a neighbor's child after school? No problem. Host the monthly moms' night in at her house because everyone else is too busy? Uh, sure. A busy mom of a toddler and a "threenager," Jill confessed that she felt overburdened and exhausted, but still couldn't shake the guilt over disappointing anyone.

It wasn't until she was asked to dog sit for a family down the street that her guilt spell was broken. She'd agreed to come over and walk their rescue hound three times a day over a long weekend. The dog barked incessantly and went crazy each time Jill showed up to let him outside. On the second day, Jill had to bring her kids along for the chore. She asked them to stay by the door, but once she released the dog, all hell broke loose—he lunged out of the crate, and her daughter screamed in fear. Jill knew the poor pup was just cooped up and anxious without his family, but the chaos freaked her out as much as it did her kids. She needed to feel that reaction to know she should have said no. One month later the same family asked for the same favor, and Jill was able to politely but firmly say, "I'm sorry, but I'm not available this weekend."

Flow Mamas can also benefit from incorporating more of their Vulnerability expression to help tap into their inner feelings and express them in constructive ways. Vulnerable Mamas are good at sharing their worries and fears, and asking for help when they need it. This kind of openness is great for Flow Mamas to practice being more in tune with their own convictions. This expression can really help Flow Mamas acknowledge and express their needs and conquer the fear of feeling like a burden simply for having needs in the first place!

Flow Mamas can also take a cue from Action Mamas' ability to create structure and set guidelines. By initiating plans instead of always following them, you'll encourage yourself to put your preferences out there and show others you're capable of setting goals and executing them. For example, maybe you arrange a weekend playdate for your kids instead of waiting for the other moms to set it up. Pick the time and place that works best for you and see if that's good for the group—you can always be flexible once you've put it out there. Once there's a plan, the work is done! You just have to show up.

ayurvedic practice for flow mamas

Ayurveda is a five-thousand-year-old medical system from India translating to the "science of life" and "knowledge of living." This Eastern modality is based on the five elements: fire, water, earth, air, and space. Each of us has all five elements that make up our being, but how much of each element and what we are mostly made of is decided at the moment of conception and constitutes our *dosha*, or mind-body type. The three doshas are Vata—air and space, Pitta—fire and water, and Kapha—earth and water. Martha Soffer and Aleiela Quintero-Allen have created this Ayurvedic practice for Flow Mamas, but any mama can use it to create greater balance in her life.

The Flow Mama is a combination of Vata and Kapha. She is very stable, creative, and grounded when in balance, but when out of balance she can lose sense of her center. Some herbs that she can take internally or infused in oil for topical use are ashwagandha, brahmi, and bacopa. These herbs will not only calm her mind but also give her the strength to speak her truth. Sandalwood and tea tree oil (mixed with a carrier oil) will also help strengthen and open the throat chakra.

> DAILY ROUTINE:

- *Wake up before 6 a.m.*
- *Dry brush your skin.*
- *Engage in regular exercise or an activity.*
- *Take daily or weekly walks outdoors in the sunlight.*
- *Keep food light, avoiding excess dairy and sweets.*
- *Eat raw fruits and vegetables only in the summer and cooked in the winter.*
- *Favor beans and legumes over red meat.*
- *Reduce sweet, salty, and sour foods.*
- *Incorporate strong spices such as cinnamon, ginger, black pepper, mustard, cumin, and turmeric.*
- *Drink tea blended with cinnamon sticks, fresh ginger, and turmeric.*

✳ NO MEANS NO—OR DOES IT?

Lucy was initially excited to meet Sarah at their girls' preschool. Both moms were easygoing and enjoyed each other's company so much they started grabbing coffee after morning drop-off. One day Sarah asked if Lucy could handle pickup that afternoon because she had a hair appointment. Lucy thought the timing was a little weird—she always booked personal appointments during school hours—but she felt bad for judging Sarah and smiled. "Sure, of course!" A similar request came a week later, and pretty soon, Lucy was driving Sarah's daughter home at least twice a week. She felt completely trapped and annoyed at herself for creating the cycle in the first place.

One morning over coffee, when Sarah asked, "Oh, you can do pickup today, right? I have to meet a client this afternoon," Lucy tried to channel her inner Action Mama and set a boundary. She started out, "Um, well, today we have to stop by the grocery store after school." It wasn't quite yes, but it wasn't quite no, either. And Lucy ended up bringing both kids to the store.

This is how Flow Mamas are easily taken advantage of. The perceived immediate pain of confrontation feels greater than the long-term pain of becoming a martyr. You may think you're drawing a line in the sand, but your body language or communication style isn't clear enough. One strategy is to come up with language that's strong enough to convey your true intent but still something you feel comfortable saying—nobody expects you to take it to code red and scream profanities (frankly, that's just rude!). But you do need to make sure your game plan is solid. Practice with a close friend you trust; a Rebel or Action Mama would be a great partner for this exercise. Pretend they've asked you for a favor, and you turn them down. Ask your buddy to be brutally honest about whether your response is clear enough. And ask yourself what feelings come up for you when you say no. If you're at a loss, check out some suggested go-to phrases at right for ideas.

the language of *no*

Saying no should be direct and clear, but it doesn't have to be rude or mean. If it helps, you can start out with something positive and genuine to help soften the blow. Just be sure, especially if you feel as if you're being put on the spot or pushed, that you repeat your polite decline until it is heard. Sometimes it's helpful to have a few go-to phrases on hand that you're comfortable with. Here are a few basic examples that you can tweak to be your own.

- "I wish I could help you, but I'm not available on that day."

- "I would love to get the kids together, but this weekend doesn't work for us. How about I suggest a few alternatives?"

- "That's a lovely offer, but we have enough backyard toys, thank you."

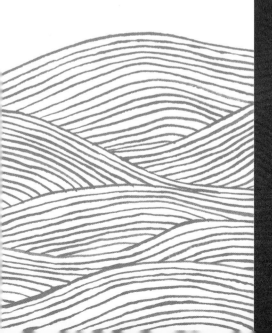

* DON'T GET TOO ATTACHED

The root of suffering is attachment.

—THE BUDDHA

To be more empowered and true to yourself, connect with your inner Free Mama and practice the art of nonattachment. Set boundaries and then practice nonattachment to the outcome. Next time you catch yourself about to say yes when your whole being is screaming, *Hell NO!*—STOP—and channel your inner Free Mama in order to worry less about what others think, take a stand, and follow through. By detaching yourself from others' reactions or judgments, you can ease away from the need to people-please, and focus instead on your own inner intuition and speak up for what you need.

Gina is a Free Mama living in her own big, beautiful world. She has no problem asking for what she wants (or saying no) because she is detached from the outcome—put simply, she never feels she has anything to lose by putting herself out there. One of Gina's friends, Wendy, an Action Mama, was organizing a school auction, and she asked Gina if she could solicit donations. Gina immediately said, "Sure!" A few weeks later, Gina walked in with the most incredible items, from a ski weekend in Aspen to a famous rock legend's signed guitar to the chance to throw the first pitch at a Major League Baseball game, and TONS more. All the other parents couldn't believe it. "How did you pull this off?"

And Gina replied, "I called and asked."

Because Gina wasn't super-attached to the outcome, her worst-case scenario was that someone might say no. Her natural sense of nonattachment was a huge win for the school!

EXERCISE:
ridiculous requests

A great way to practice nonattachment is to play a game where you make ridiculous requests, knowing that they are so impossible, the answer will probably be no.

For one month, each day you'll make a Ridiculous Request. The purpose of this exercise is not to collect a ton of yeses based on your Ridiculous Request; rather the purpose is in the asking itself. It's a way to exercise the muscle of asking and have no expectations. The best part is that whether you get a yes or no, you win! When you ask something ridiculous, you don't expect that someone will say yes. This way, you are pleasantly surprised when they do. If you don't ask, you'll never know. #winning

A Ridiculous Request can be as simple as asking for a free coffee to something more extravagant. My friend Kristen originally intended to ask for a business class upgrade on her overnight flight, but then thought, *Well, if I'm gonna ask, I might as well go big or go home!* She asked for a first-class upgrade and the ticket agent said, "YES!" Kristen grinned all the way from LA to New York City with a big glass of Pinot Noir and her latest juicy novel, enjoying a much-needed spoiling (she is the single mom to a very active nine-year-old).

If you never ask, you'll never know. And life's too short to sit around always wondering what could have been.

* KNOW WHEN TO SAY NO— AND STILL KEEP YOUR FLOW

Saying no can be one of the hardest things for *anyone* to do. But the benefits of setting boundaries are huge. You may be surprised to find that once you let people know what works for you and where you stand, they respect you more for it. Not to mention you will have a lot more energy and space for the things you want to say yes to.

So how do you know when to say no when your whole body feels wired to be agreeable all the time? It comes back to being able to tap into your intuition. If you're asked to do something and it makes you feel uncomfortable or uneasy, there's a reason for that—it's probably not something you really want or feel able to do. This feeling can manifest in various physical ways: your shoulders hunch up, you grit your teeth, your jaw tightens, you feel a tightness in your stomach, or you make a simple internal *ugh* or an eye roll. Many of us get these internal signals because our gut instinct knows we should say NO! but we ignore the message and go on with a tentative smile and say yes.

Flow Mamas can practice setting simple boundaries in order to check in with their truth and understand their own preferences. Perhaps it's as basic as saying a cheerful "No thanks" to the juice rep in the grocery store offering free samples (be honest, maybe it's your least favorite flavor). Work up to bigger challenges, such as turning down a playdate that doesn't work for your schedule. You may even find that you create a better relationship once you are able to say no and let people know what works for you. Believe in yourself and what you have to offer.

the human pendulum

I attended a lecture last year that Alessandro Giannotti, a healer and spiritual teacher, taught on intuition, and he shared the following exercise. He had us all stand up and close our eyes and think of two choices we were considering making. We had to imagine that one was in front of us and the other behind. And then he had us meditate on the choices. After a few moments he had us stop where we were and asked us to take note on which way our bodies were leaning. That was our intuition guiding us. I practice this often and share it with all my mamas when they aren't sure which choice to make.

Stand tall and strong with your feet flat on the floor and your arms by your sides. Close your eyes and think of two very simple choices: Pizza or pasta? Jeans or a dress? Go out or stay in? Picture one choice in front of you, and one choice behind you. Now imagine a pendulum swinging forward and backward between both choices and notice how your body reacts. Do you feel like you are gravitating toward the front or toward the back? Does your body actually start swaying? Use your body and instincts instead of your head, and pay attention to where your energy naturally flows. Even if both choices seem fine, I'm willing to bet you'll end up on one side. The whole goal of this exercise is not to overthink it! You'll practice a further deepening of your own intuition and making choices for yourself.

By strengthening her own convictions, the Flow Mama can continue to share her valuable gift of flexibility, knowing she can speak up for herself when she needs to.

Your easygoing, flowing nature makes you an ideal partner, *most* of the time. Your challenge is to overcome your fear of confrontation and chaos, and stand in your own convictions, no matter how it plays out. Know that certain people can't or won't hear you and others may react negatively when you set boundaries or stand up for yourself. Practice letting go of your attachment to outcome so you won't fear the worst. By tapping into the other expressions, you can strengthen your sense of self-protection, freedom to speak your truth, and confidence to live in the present moment.

flow mama toolkit

✳ Flow Recipe:
Red Dates, Goji, and Loganberry Tea

You put all your energy toward others, often at the expense of your own health and wellness. Heng Ou crafted this recipe with red dates to combat insomnia and loganberries to soothe stress and anxiety, helping bring you back into your body so you can tap into what *you* need.

SERVES 4–5

- *2 whole dried red dates*
- *4 whole dried loganberries*
- *1 teaspoon dried goji berries*

➤ Bring 6 cups (1400 ml) water to a boil in a medium pot. Halve the red dates and add them to the boiling water. Lower the heat to a simmer and cook for 45 minutes, uncovered. In the last 20 minutes, add the loganberries and goji berries. The red dates and loganberries provide enough sweetness, so I normally leave extra sweetener out.

➤ Strain and sip throughout the day or store in the fridge for up to 1 week.

✳ Flow Supplements:
Find Your Fire

Elissa Goodman recommends these nutritional supplements to balance your system and give your body a boost where it needs it most.

Gaia Maca: This root helps increase energy so you can feel more motivated to take charge

Pure Encapsulations L-Tyrosine: L-Tyrosine is an amino acid that is used to boost focus and clarity.

Hawaiian Spirulina: This supplement helps increase energy and strength to take on anything!

✳ Flow Oils:
Stay Centered

All these oils can be diffused, added to a bath, or worn as a healing perfume. A lot of essential oil blends often contain hidden chemicals, so I recommend Young Living Essentials Oils for their high-grade quality and purity.

YOUNG LIVING ESSENTIAL OILS

Harmony Blend: for energy balance

Release Blend: for emotional balance

Motivation Blend: to create positive energy and forward movement

✳ Flow Crystals:
Enjoy Peace in Your Truth

When you first get your crystal, you have to solidify your bond. As with any relationship, it takes time for your energies to sync. For a crystal to purify your energy, you have to first return the gesture and cleanse its energy. You can let your crystal bathe outside in the light of the sun or moon for at least four hours, or place it on the soil or hang it on the branch of a healthy houseplant for twenty-four hours. Then sit quietly, holding the stone in both your hands. Visualize your intention for the crystal. The stone is listening. Giving your crystal a job allows you to set your intention for the work you'll do together. It's okay to get specific! After programming the crystal with your intention, your crystal is now activated. Heather Askinosie has chosen these crystals specifically to help Flow Mamas find their inner truth.

Andalusite: This stone will help Flow Mamas establish clear boundaries. When Flow Mamas fall into the negative habit of accommodating everyone but themselves, they can tune into andalusite's protective energy. It will encourage them to be fluid with their truth, so that they have the confidence to express themselves and say no when they need to. Embracing andalusite energy will bring Flow Mamas to understand and harness their personal power, so that they remember to honor themselves as a priority.

Pink Opal: Peace and tranquility is where the energy of fluidity lives. As the Flow Mama finds strength in knowing that she must respect her own needs as well as others, she can find true fluidity with pink opal. Often we can mistake resigning to the will of others and silently resenting it as going with the flow. Pink opal energy connects to the heart chakra to flood it with strength, love, forgiveness, and joy. The energy of resentments keeps you mentally and emotionally stuck in a certain situation. Pink opal will help you forgive and move past it, as well as provide the self-loving strength to assert your needs in the future.

flow yoga:
stand strong in your truth

~~~~~~~~~~~~~~~~~~~~~~~~~~~~~~~

This yoga sequence will help you find your center and activate your voice. These poses are designed to activate your third and fifth chakras (power and communication center) to help you find your truth, stand strong in it, and express it.

Suggested props: mat, 2 yoga blocks, bolster, timer

✳ Supported Mid Back Bend with Blocks

- Place one block horizontal under your mid back with your diaphragm area on the medium height of the block. Place the other block vertically under the back of your head for support. Legs can be crossed on the floor, extended out straight, or bent with feet flat on the floor and knees up.

- Focus your attention on your diaphragm area, which is located in the lower front of your rib cage. Imagine a big yellow balloon hovering above this area of your body. As you breathe in through your nose, see the yellow balloon going into your diaphragm. As you exhale through your nose, visualize that yellow balloon going out. Keep this going for 1 to 3 minutes. As you breathe in, see that yellow color expanding within, and when you breathe out, see it extending out further.

❋ Gentle Twist

- Lying on your back, set the blocks aside and hug your knees into your chest.

- Bring both knees across the left side of your body to the ground and look to the right. Imagine your breath as a magical healing tool and tint it with the color of sunlight. Breathe into any tightness as if you are breathing in the light, and as you exhale, soften and relax this area as you breathe out any darkness. Take 6 slow and deep breaths like this. Switch sides and repeat.

❋ Supported Cobra to Plank

- Hug your knees back into your chest and then roll over onto your belly.

- Place your hands flat on floor. As you inhale through your nose, straighten your arms and lift your torso off the ground. Bend your elbows and exhale out of your mouth as you lower your torso down to the ground. Right away come up and then come down, linking your breath with your movement, and each time you come down, turn your head, alternating from right to left. Repeat 10 times.

- Lift your hips off the ground to come up to plank and hold for 1 minute.

- Come back to the ground and repeat up and down cobra 10 times.

- Come up to plank and hold for 1 minute.

- Come back to the ground and repeat up and down cobra 10 times.

- Come up to plank and hold for 1 minute.

✳ Bow

- Come down to the ground.

- Lying with your belly flat on the ground, reach your arms out in front. Inhale and lift just your arms and torso off the ground, leaving your legs on the floor. Take 3 deep, slow breaths. Come down and relax.

- Reach your arms out to the side and lift your torso, legs still on the ground. Hold and breathe for 3 slow counts.

- Do the same thing again, but this time with your arms clasped behind your back. Hold, legs still on the ground, and breathe 3 slow breaths.

- Reach behind you, bend your knees, and grab your ankles. Inhale and lift your torso up, pushing your feet slowly toward the back of the room. Hold for 3 breaths and then come down to rest. Repeat 3 times.

✳ Child's Pose

- Begin on your hands and knees and spread your knees apart, with your big toes touching.
- Take a deep breath and bow forward, so your torso is between your thighs. Allow your forehead to come to the floor.
- Gently sway forward and backward.

✳ Torso Rolls

- Come up into a cross-legged position. Place your hands on your knees. Move your torso in a circle clockwise for 1 to 3 minutes. Then change directions. This will stir up energy in the third chakra.

✳ Seated Cat/Cow

- Imagine a bright yellow flame in your third chakra area. Every time you inhale, you stoke the fire, breathing away anything that's blocking you from stepping into your power. Every time you exhale, you breathe out the dark ashes of what no longer serves you. Still in a cross-legged position, place your hands on your ankles. Inhale through your nose, stoking the fire, arch, and look up. Exhale the ashes of what needs to go through your mouth as you drop your head and round your back while you pull back.

✳ Seated Twist

- Still in a cross-legged position, place your right hand on your left knee and reach your left hand to the ground slightly behind your left hip. Take 5 deep breaths. Switch sides and repeat.

✳ Shoulder Shrugs with Lion's Breath

- Raise your shoulders up toward your ears. Exhale strongly through your mouth while you quickly drop your shoulders down, making a "ha" sound. As you exhale, open your mouth wide and stick your tongue out as far as possible toward your chin. Repeat 3 times. Each time, think of releasing something that you wanted to say but didn't, or imagine any anger or resentment you felt because you allowed a boundary to be crossed or didn't take a stance for your truth.

✳ Neck Rolls

- Roll your neck, 5 times to the left and 5 times to the right.

✳ Neck Stretch

- Place your right hand by the top of your left ear, gently pulling your head toward your right shoulder. Walk your left hand to the left side on the ground, inhale into the left side of your neck, and as you exhale, allow your right shoulder to drop. Do 5 deep, slow breaths and then repeat on the other side.

✳ Jaw Massage

- Place the top of your thumbs on the sides of your face where your jaw hinges. Open and close and feel for a slight dip. When you find it, inhale and, when you exhale, apply firm pressure as you allow your jaw to open and relax. Keep doing this a few times. Then, take your knuckles and massage around your whole jaw area.

✳ Chanting

- Set a timer for 11 minutes. Place the root (not the tip) of your tongue on the roof of your mouth and tuck your chin down. Chant this out loud: *Humee Hum Brahm Hums*. (You can download this chant on iTunes.) The yogi and spiritual teacher Yogi Bhajan, who introduced Kundalini Yoga to the United States, encouraged this practice to stimulate the throat chakra. You may think you sound ridiculous and the chant is REALLY hard to say, but trust me, you'll be killing it with your throat chakra when you're done with this.

✳ Speak Your Truth Visualization

- Call back your power by visualizing speaking your truth.

- Place a spine-length bolster at your butt and lie back, legs straight out on the floor. Inhale, just like how you started in the first posture with the yellow balloon. This time breathe the yellow balloon into your diaphragm area and visualize it traveling up. As it does, it changes color to blue. Breathe the blue out from your throat. Do this for a few rounds.

- Think about something that happened where you didn't speak your truth or you gave your power away to someone else. When you get an image, see them sitting across from you facing you. Imagine all the power you gave away in their belly as yellow light, and as you inhale, breathe it back into your own power center as if you are vacuuming it back to where it belongs. As you exhale, breathe out through your mouth blue energy—all the things you didn't say but wanted to. Keep breathing in, taking back your power, and breathing out your truth that wasn't spoken.

- When you have nothing more to take back or speak, sit up in a cross-legged position and bring your hands into prayer. Take a moment to set an intention to create boundaries when and where needed and to work on speaking your truth even if your voice shakes.

flow affirmations:
speak out

Practice saying one or more of these phrases that resonate with you by speaking them to yourself in a mirror once a day, or write them down and stick them somewhere you'll see them daily. You may not feel comfortable at first, but over time, by repeating these affirmations out loud, or writing them out over and over, you'll reinforce your resilience and ability to stand strong in your own truth.

IT'S OKAY TO SAY NO.

I ALWAYS HAVE A CHOICE.

MY NEEDS ARE IMPORTANT.

I CAN'T PLEASE EVERYONE.

I CAN BE A KIND PERSON WITH A GOOD HEART
AND STILL SAY NO.

"NO" IS A COMPLETE SENTENCE.

I AM ALLOWED TO SPEAK UP FOR WHAT I BELIEVE IN.

MY OPINION MATTERS.

I SPEAK MY TRUTH WITH EASE.

IT'S OKAY NOT TO AGREE WITH OR DO
WHAT OTHERS ARE DOING.

I STAND STRONG IN MY TRUTH.

I TRUST MYSELF.

I AM NOT RESPONSIBLE FOR
PLEASING EVERYONE.

flow meditation:
honor yourself

The ability to flow with other people and outer circumstances is a great gift. Taken too far, or when we lose our own "individual flow," we tend to not get our own needs met and begin to lose touch with our "inner self," "inner knowing," and feelings. We become what Michele Meiche calls "too merge-y." We merge with everyone and everything else and lose track of ourselves.

Understanding that we are an important part of our own life (and including our needs into relationships) is a key learning lesson. It is also very empowering, as well as a form of self-love.

Being able to get along with others, take the high road, and put others' needs above our own are very good personality traits. They reflect empathy as well as an ability to care for and really be there for others. The healing and empowering balancing point is to integrate an acknowledgment of your own feelings and life needs. This means it's important that you learn to recognize, feel, and honor your own individual flow.

Do this Mindful Moment Meditation by Michele Meiche daily for ninety days, and then as needed. It takes about this amount of time to integrate a new pattern of behavior. Think of it as your "personal healing and empowerment guarantee." I suggest doing this meditation to start your day. This will help you discern your true needs and priorities. This meditation will assist you and support you in connecting more to your intuition, as well as provide an inner knowing of what is right for you. Ultimately, what is right for you will be right for your baby, family, friends, etc.

You can do this with your eyes open or closed. If your eyes are open, it is best to have them slightly closed, relaxed, and looking down toward the floor. This is to heighten your awareness as to what is going on inside you while you are still focused on outer concerns and the people in your life. This trains you to do both more easily and consistently.

Stand with your feet hip-width apart, with your legs slightly bent. It is best not to lock your knees.

Think of where you are, the people in your life, and what you have to do for your day.

Take a deep breath in, and as you breathe out, scan your body. Become aware of how you are feeling.

Notice how you are feeling in your body.

Notice any areas of tightness.

Notice any areas that you tend to feel more.

Notice any areas that you are not normally aware of, or that you don't normally feel.

Breathe in and slightly pause your breath. This centers you inside.

Breathe out and feel the feelings in your body.

Notice how when you breathe out you become more aware of your body and the feelings within your body.

Now breathe in a little slower.

Pause your breath as you center inside.

Breathe out a little slower as you become more aware of your body and what you are feeling.

Breathe in a little slower.

Pause your breath slightly as you center inside.

Breathe out a little slower as you become more aware of your body and how you are feeling.

Breathe in a little slower.

Pause your breath slightly as you center inside.

Breathe out a little slower as you become more aware of your body and how you are feeling.

Now ask yourself in your own mind and own way what you feel like doing and what you actually need to do.

Keep your focus on your breath as you get your own answer from within.

This answer may come in a flash of insight, a word, a feeling, or even the face of someone you need to call.

Trust the messages and guidance you receive from within.

This will help you align to your own individual flow and prioritize.

The more you do this Mindful Moment Meditation, the more you will create an inner balance inside. This will allow you to know what you have the energy, emotional capacity, and mind-set to do. When you prioritize from this perspective, you will get more done in less time, and perhaps come to see so much of what you did in the past that you actually didn't need to do.

deepening your self-awareness

Answer these questions in order, as they build upon each other, to continue understanding and connecting with your inner Flow Mama expression:

1. Where does or where has your Flow expression shown up in your life?

2. What do you resist or find most off-putting about Flow Mamas?

3. Where do you resist this aspect of the Flow Mama within yourself?

4. Who's your favorite Flow Mama and what do you admire about her?

5. Where can you see parts of her reflected in you?

6. How might your life change from integrating more of your Flow expression into your life and being?

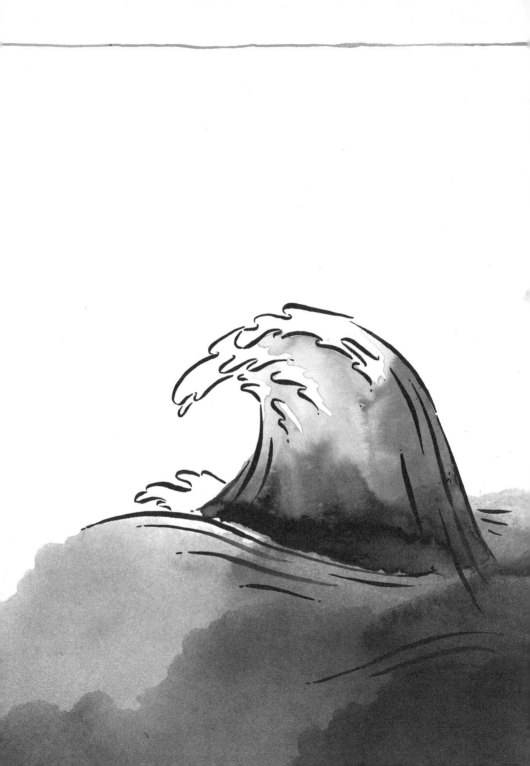

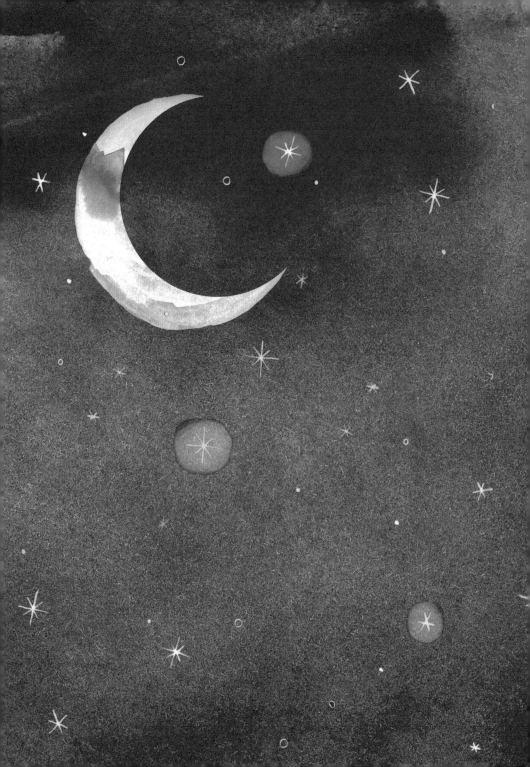

chapter five

REBEL MAMA

Born to Be Wild

〜〜〜〜〜〜〜〜〜〜〜〜〜〜

Hey there, Rebel Mama. I'm aware that you don't want my advice. I get it. In fact, even just the *idea* of advice makes you run screaming in the opposite direction. You are a one-of-a-kind, original badass who isn't afraid to express your truth and authenticity in anything you do. You're usually blazing new trails while marching to the beat of your own drum—your vibe is more freewheeling and spontaneous than perfectly pulled together—and you never hesitate to stand up for what you believe in even if you stand alone. Why should you give a shit what anyone else thinks of you? Your independence and confidence are what give you strength.

Trust me, I'm not going to tell you what to do. If anyone tries to force authority on you, it'll probably blow up in their face! I get that you don't like feeling rushed or pushed in any direction. I'm just going to plant a few seeds of information for you to grow in your own way and your own time. I respect that you need time to process and feel free to make your own choices. I've had so much success working with my Rebel Mamas using this approach—by giving them the space to develop their own path forward, I see them blossom in their own unique and beautifully rebellious way.

Let's be honest. Parenting can be mundane. And that's the furthest thing from what interests you. A lot of Rebel Mamas possess a highly creative and artistic drive. Coloring outside the lines isn't enough—you want to color all over the walls! Rebel Mamas often create from their own emotions and experiences, and translate their inner vision through music, art, literature, design, and more. You have a broad view of the world and aren't afraid to explore new realms, bringing others along with you. Following the rules makes you cringe, but because you insist on doing everything your own way, you may not be as willing to adopt a routine or conform to any structure. And that can be challenging as a mom, given all the things that happen on a daily basis: meals, naps, playdates, activities, bedtime. How can you surrender to "the norm" without feeling restricted?

Rebel Mamas can tap into their inner Action Mama when it comes to the basics—sticking to a schedule but softening the lines so it still feels spontaneous and fun. For example, you might shake up dinnertime by letting your kids choose what's for dinner and help you cook (in other words, guaranteed chaos). Or, maybe you invite friends or neighbors over last-minute to join in the fun. I wouldn't be surprised if you packed a picnic and had dinner in a teepee in your backyard!

✳ REBEL WITHOUT A CAUSE

Others may surrender to authority easily or accept the status quo without question (it drives you crazy, I know!), but you prefer to be independent. That's okay, as long as you're not getting stuck in your own stubborn streak. Embracing your inner Flow Mama can help you stay flexible in your approach. Flow Mamas are so named because they are usually content to take a back seat and let other people drive the train. They're happy to go along with others' rules or preferences as long as it keeps the group copacetic and the energy positive. Rebels can channel their inner Flow expression to help allow for new ideas and trust that the universe is on their side. (This works both ways: Flow Mamas can channel a bit more of their inner Rebel Mamas' defiance when they want to assert themselves.) Integrating their inner Free Mama expression further helps Rebel Mamas release their attachment to outcome. I'll be the first to admit this isn't easy—it's something our Buddhist friends spend a lifetime aspiring to achieve!

One of my clients, Josie, reluctantly signed up for a toddler music class. Her girlfriend assured her that it wasn't the typical kind of group, because there's no way she was gonna sit through an hour of Ring around the Rosy! Ten minutes into the first class, her son threw an epic temper tantrum. The well-meaning teacher quickly offered some advice, which made Josie feel defensive. "I got it," she said bluntly, even as her son continued screaming on the floor.

She had to force herself to go back to the class the next week. As the music started, another little girl began having a meltdown. Josie watched as the toddler's mom used the advice the teacher had given the week before. Soon enough, the toddler calmed down and the music continued, and Josie realized it might be worth trying a new technique. Within days, her son stopped his defiant behavior, and Josie admitted that being more flexible and listening to others wasn't such a bad idea.

When you find yourself pushing back against someone's suggestion or doubling down on your stance, ask yourself if you're doing it because you're *really* that passionate, or if it's just because you're feeling pressured. If it's the latter, how could you ask for some space to make up your own mind? Another way to create space is to tap into your inner Free Mama in order to detach from what's going on in the moment and adopt a more neutral perspective. With some practice, you can literally distance yourself by observing both yourself and the scene around you from above.

EXERCISE:
how to pause

Rebels tend to be reactive. Learning to pause instead of reacting or, conversely, shutting down, will help you become more receptive and compassionate. Try the following exercise the next time you feel your energy rising up, when you are about to lash out, push back, or shut off. In other words, it's the feeling you get right before you're about to tell someone to get lost!

Everybody's trigger indications are different, depending on the person and situation, but most people share some common physical sensations. Indications are things such as (but certainly not limited to): gritting your teeth, tightness in your jaw, holding your breath, becoming fidgety, a headache or pounding in your head, feeling agitated and irritable, getting hot or red in the face. Learning to recognize these physical triggers can help you know when to practice the pause. Trust me, reacting may feel good short-term, but this method will allow you to soften your demeanor, take the edge off, and conserve your energy for more positive activities.

- When you feel physically triggered, that's your cue to STOP.

- Take a deep breath (or up to 100 deep breaths if you need to).

- Feel your feet planted firmly on the ground.

- Feel your energy rise above you. Imagine you are watching the situation from above, and become a detached observer.

- As you detach from yourself and look at what's triggering you, try to understand the situation as if it's happening to someone else. In other words, try to see it from an objective perspective. Look from a higher place of empathy, compassion, and self-awareness (i.e. from a different perspective).

- Ask yourself these questions: "What is it about this person or situation that has me feeling all triggered?" "Am I really that passionate, or am I resisting something because I'm feeling pressured or resisting authority?" "Could it be possible that they might be trying to help me or have something useful to say?"

- As you translate the situation with a more empathetic, self-aware perspective, bring yourself back and try to communicate as a detached observer. You will feel more level-headed and able to express yourself more clearly so that you can be heard.

Pausing to take yourself out of the situation will make you less reactive and able to see it from another point of view.

✳ RECONNECT WITH YOUR INNER CHILD

I spoke a lot about the inner child in my previous book, *The Mindful Mom-to-Be*. When you embrace and reconnect with your own inner child, you will be less likely to try to re-create your lost childhood through your children. Now, Rebel Mama, I know you love to do things outside the box and you have no problem allowing and encouraging your children to do the same. But in order to have a fuller, more empathetic relationship with your children (or anyone, for that matter), it's important to have a relationship with your inner child and reconnect with, find, and embrace your own innocence.

My client Betsy was having a hard time being patient with her child's temper tantrums, nonstop questions, and emotional reactions to things she felt were meaningless. I asked her what her childhood was like, and she said her parents weren't physically or emotionally available. Her dad traveled nonstop and her mom worked two jobs, and they struggled with alcoholism and later divorced. All this caused Betsy to grow up way too fast and fend for herself. I asked Betsy to do the exercise on page 104 to help reclaim her innocence. This is something I do with many of my clients when I feel they need to reconnect and reintegrate a lost part of themselves.

Over the years I've worked with various shamans who talk about the times in our lives where our soul splits. We need to go back beyond an event that happened to recapture what we lost, because what we lost is what we need to integrate into our lives now. Therein lies our innocence. In order to heal, we must go back to the turning point so we can experience again where we were just before that crucial experience. We can't begin the healing process unless there is an awareness of where the wounding first started. This is an especially important exercise for Rebels. It can be extra-challenging to relate to young children if you can't tap into your own innocence.

✳ ALL MAMAS NEED A REBEL YELL

In today's social media–dominated world, moms often relentlessly compare and compete with each other. It's hard not to swipe through the rosy-filtered "reality" of perfect-looking outfits, vacations, or birthday parties and not feel even a *tiny* bit of envy. But even despite this intense pressure, Rebel Mamas typically still don't give a shit what anyone thinks of them (or what they're posting on Instagram!). A Rebel Mama is all about putting herself out there in her own unique way.

This true freedom of expression is the perfect rebel energy for any mama to channel. Action Mamas, when you feel too restricted by routine or trapped in a self-made cage of perfection, let out some steam by coloring outside the lines and breaking some of your own rules. It can be as simple as letting your kids wear whatever they want to school one day—yes, *anything*. If it makes you cringe when your son trots off to his classroom in pajama pants and a superhero cape, that's good! It means you're stretching yourself beyond your comfort zone to practice letting go of your need to appear in control 100 percent of the time.

Flow Mamas can also greatly benefit from channeling rebel energy. Kristen was so laid-back, she often let it go when her kids encountered issues on the playground. If they were pushed or teased, she sat back passively, assuming the kids would work it

reclaim your innocence

Get into a comfortable seated position. Feel the ground beneath you and take in all your surroundings. Feel the air on your skin, sense the smell in the air, listen to the sounds, and see all the sights around you that are right here and right now in this moment.

Visualize your life as if your thoughts, experiences, and emotions were projected onto a big movie screen in front of you. Start in the present moment and go backward through time to your earliest memories, perhaps the point in your childhood when you felt the most innocent and carefree. Breathe that experience into your body and breathe out any hard, rough energy. Notice what's happening in your body at that moment. Capture this place using the following questions:

- Where are you?
- Who are you with?
- How old are you?
- What do you look like?
- What are you wearing?

- What are you doing?
- How are you feeling?
- What do you need?
- What are your wishes?
- Who are you?

In order to deepen this practice, it's important to share freely without thinking too hard or editing yourself—some of my clients prefer to type out their responses or even use talk-to-text because it allows them to put their feelings out there quickly and easily.

Now choose three words that really capture the essence of who you were and how you felt at this time. When my client Betsy did this exercise, she pulled her three words from a sentence she wrote as part of her longer journal entry:

I am playing and running around barefoot outside catching lightning bugs with my brother. We are laughing, feeling totally **happy**, **carefree**, and **safe**. Summertime is the best!

I then asked Betsy: Consider how you could integrate these three words into your life today. Think about what you may have left behind in your childhood that you would like to bring with you now. What do you need that you are not getting?

For Betsy, it was obvious that her parents' divorce caused the soul split that left her feeling lost and alone. She developed newfound strength and resilience, but it came with a hardness and rigidity. She existed this way for so long, it took a while for her to acknowledge that she wished she could feel happier and more carefree around her kids. She couldn't change the past, but she could push beyond the split to reclaim an important part of her true nature.

The premise of this book is that when you connect with all the parts of yourself, you start to see yourself in others and lose the need to judge or compare. *The mother in me honors the mother in you. I am you and you are me and we are one.* This is true of mothers, women, and all people, including your children. Living in *Mamaste* allows you to tap into and reclaim parts of your essence that you might have lost that your children are reflecting back to you.

out on their own or that another parent would step in and handle the situation. But one day, she discovered her son was one of four children being bullied at school. The school called a meeting, and she found herself having a heated conversation in a room with several other concerned mothers. A mom stood up and cried, "My son is being *hurt*! This is not okay." Suddenly, Kristen felt her stomach tighten. Nobody messes with her baby, either! Being a people pleaser took a backseat to her son's welfare, and she felt a surge of inner mama bear strength rise within her. By igniting her inner rebel fire, she could stand strong in her own conviction and do whatever was necessary to support and protect her son.

A little rebel energy can greatly benefit Free Mamas, too, by igniting a sense of passion and depth and connecting to themselves and the world around them. As all mamas know, nothing brings you crashing down to earth more than having a child! When a Free Mama finds herself taking a nosedive, embracing her inner Rebel Mama might just make the landing a whole lot easier.

Jasmine struggled with adversity, preferring always to choose a plan B rather than deal with reality. Then her second son was born with developmental delays. When it came time for him to attend school, there was no plan B. She had to show up and DEAL with everything from early intervention services to getting him integrated back into general education classrooms. Jasmine channeled her inner Rebel for her baby because she knew no one else would.

All mamas have an inner Rebel, or "mama bear," as some like to say. The transformative process of becoming a mother can often ignite a fiery passion inside you and give you the courage to take a stand when you need to. Don't be afraid of this power! Learn to harness it for the good of your family.

*TRANSFORM EMOTIONS INTO ART

Many Rebel Mamas I have worked with are creative geniuses—whether or not they are paid to perform! They feel deeply, and often need to detach from their own emotions (like Free Mamas) because they feel so much. We all know what happens when we keep our emotions bottled up inside for too long—eventually, we explode. Being creative is a constructive way for a Rebel Mama to express herself and release some of that emotional pressure. I just think of artists like Beyoncé, and how she's able to translate her emotional energy into music that blows all of our freakin' minds! There may be only one Beyoncé, but there's also only one of *you*.

I worked with a Rebel Mama who needed a creative way to process her emotions and feelings about a past birth experience. With her first pregnancy, she had planned for a natural birth but ended up having a caesarian due to placenta previa (a condition where the placenta completely covers the cervix). She'd had a rough recovery and was disappointed in the whole experience. Now she was planning a VBAC (vaginal birth after caesarian) for her second child. Because she was really struggling and holding on to the past, we agreed to find a way to help her process and clear the negative memories from her first pregnancy and delivery. I didn't want anything to get in the way of her upcoming birth experience.

She wasn't an artist, but I asked her to come up with a piece of artwork to represent her past feelings. I assured her it was for her eyes only, the goal being to transform emotions into inspiration and shed her body of lingering negativity. She decided to buy a set of paints and a canvas, and I really credit her for going for it—she took the assignment to heart and created an incredible piece of modern artwork that spoke about her journey. It shared everything, from the birth she had hoped for, to the scar from the caesarean, to the immediate love for her newborn baby, to the disappointment, fear, and anger she felt that her body didn't cooperate the way she had intended. Her artwork was authentic, and it freed her up to move on and embrace a new beginning. The piece is hanging in her bathroom, and she now paints regularly as an act of self-care to help her move her energy forward by transforming it into art.

If painting isn't your thing, you might want to try one of these: poetry, writing, singing, music, dancing, sculpting, acting, photography, sketching, drawing. Rebel Mamas tend to want to explore artistic pursuits on their own, but don't discount the potential fun in taking a class with a friend or two—even if you end up hysterically laughing after a busted belly-dancing class, it's still time well spent on releasing emotional energy.

✳HOW TO RELATE WHEN A REBEL RULES

Think about how small children interact with each other at the playground—they rarely "tell" each other what they're doing; they "show" each other simply by doing and following each other's leads. For Rebel Mamas, who resist any level of authority, it's critical to shift your approach so they can trust and follow you instead of resisting and battling you. When I work with my Rebel Mamas, I like to "plant seeds" by simply sharing stories, not giving advice. Speaking from a place of sharing and storytelling is a great way to communicate with Rebel Mamas. Instead of suggesting, "You should try an art class," try something like, "I went to this amazing art class with my kids, and we used elements in nature to create collages—it was so fun! We learned all about local plants." If your Rebel Mama is interested, she may start asking questions or just sign up for the next class. Or she may invite you over for a nature class in her own backyard! Rebel Mamas do well with this kind of seed-planting, and letting those seeds sprout in their own time and way.

Jackie, one of my Action Mamas, had signed up for a Mommy and Me yoga class at my suggestion. She really struggled with perfectionism and constantly worried whether she was doing the right thing. I thought yoga would help her invite openness into her life. In the first class, as she settled in with her baby, mat, and blankets, she noticed a woman walk in with a presence that turned everyone's heads. Sasha, a true Rebel Mama, strode into the room wearing pajama bottoms and a mismatched top, with blue streaks in her messy topknot. She plopped down on the floor with her baby (wearing just a diaper) and whipped out her boob to nurse. Jackie was horrified. *Who goes out in public like that? It may be warm, but where are your baby's clothes?!*

During class, Jackie watched as Sasha expertly moved through the yoga poses with her newborn, gently and softly singing to the baby. Despite the way she looked to Jackie, she was a terrific mother, and she seemed to get more joy out of the class than anyone else. As everyone relaxed in namaste, Jackie smelled something familiar and foul—she looked over to see Sasha struggling with a massive diaper blowout. "I left my bag at home, and he already pooped all over the outfit I had him in earlier!" she whispered.

Are you kidding me? Left it at home? How irresponsible! "Judge" Jackie first thought. But then, something magical happened. She remembered when she'd forgotten something or felt overwhelmed. She offered Sasha a diaper and an extra change of clothes (of course she had packed three, just in case). Her simple act of empathy and kindness made both women smile, and they felt an unexpected connection, however momentarily, as kindred mom-spirits.

Rebels can often seem intimidating or unreachable because they stand so strongly in their own truths. But remember that they're dealing with all the same struggles and fears as any other mom; they just don't always show it in the same way. So if you feel yourself becoming threatened or rushing to judge, remember that it's always worth taking a moment to *Mamaste*. The Rebel in her is the Rebel in you. I promise you both possess this expression and the ability to channel it anytime in your own way.

*LISTEN TO THE WHISPER BEFORE IT BECOMES A SHOUT

If you are so strong in holding on to your conviction, your unwillingness to be open to looking at another point of view could potentially hurt you in the long run. You might miss out on things that have been proven to be beneficial, helpful, and make things possibly easier for you, your family, and child.

—RICHARD CRENNA, MARRIAGE AND FAMILY THERAPIST

Rebel Mamas often think in linear or polarizing terms. It can feel lonely when you trust only yourself or get backed into a corner because it's your way or the highway. Think about how this has impacted your relationships, whether with friends, your partner, or even your kids. Feeling as if you're the lone wolf against the world may spark your determination, but it's also very isolating. How could you develop some trust that others have your best interest at heart, and encourage yourself to ask for help (and accept it) when you need it?

As I like to say, listen to the whisper before it becomes a shout.

My client Briana was breastfeeding just fine when she left the hospital after giving birth, but when she got home, everything fell apart. Her friend suggested a lactation consultant who had really helped her. Briana resisted—she didn't want a stranger coming over with a new baby in the house, but truthfully, she *really* didn't like being told what to do. After clogged ducts and a bout of mastitis, in desperation, she finally reached out to the lactation specialist. Within three minutes of the visit, she learned the techniques she needed to latch properly, and it turned the entire experience around. For Briana, it took hitting bottom to admit her vulnerability. After that, she realized she didn't need to wait until things were unbearable to reach out for help.

Because your MO is to think outside the box, you also tend to roll your eyes at anything too "normal." You are *not* a basic mom! But staying open to new ideas, regardless of how they're delivered, might be the key to finding new paths you love exploring so much. So what if the seemingly traditional preschool director is the one who mentioned the pop-up flea market downtown—you went and scored the exact vintage crib you were looking for!

momspirations

Grab a small notebook to keep by your bedside. Each night, before you go to sleep, write down one thing you learned that day. It could be anything, from "momspirations" to real emotional breakthroughs, such as the following:

> Daycare pickup is so stressful, as I'm always late. I feel terrible about it, and it's costing me a fortune in late fees! Yesterday another mom invited me to join her carpool. At first I didn't want to commit to this, but it would be a great solution. Maybe I'll try it once a week and see how it goes.

> I saw a mom park at the school and go for a run in the neighborhood instead of heading back into traffic. Maybe I could try this sometime when I don't have afternoon meetings.

> We went to my son's friend's house for dinner tonight. The mother had her kids sit and eat dinner at the table. Though we don't usually do a conventional dinner, I am going to give this a shot, as it would give our family an opportunity to connect at the end of the day.

Observing others is a great way for Rebel Mamas to learn without being told what to do. It's a subtler way to receive information without risk of confrontation or resistance. Some of the best lessons my clients have learned are by secretly observing other moms they may not necessarily like or even know—inspiration is the best form of *Mamaste*.

✳ JUST SAY YES— OPENING TO RESISTANCE

Boundaries are important and Rebel Mamas are very good at setting them. Because you're so strong in your own beliefs and shed outer judgment like water off a duck, it's easier for you to draw your lines in the sand. That said, think about when your last *no* went from creating a boundary to creating a barrier. By insisting on doing things your way, you can miss out on unexpected opportunities. What if, instead of saying no, you occasionally encouraged yourself to say yes? Think about how this might open you up to a world of new possibilities.

One of my clients told me a great story: Her daughter's teacher asked her to volunteer for a class field trip to sing Christmas carols at a nursing home. Her initial response was, *Ugh, I would rather watch paint dry*, but she realized it was a chance to spend time with her daughter and do some good in the world. She reluctantly said yes and ended up having a blast with the kids *and* the old-timers. They sang only two traditional carols, then switched gears completely, singing show tunes and pop hits, dancing and laughing up a storm. She even facilitated a wheelchair race! When you open yourself up to things you may initially resist, the surprises are endless.

✳SOFTENING THE EDGES

Rebel Mamas, believe it or not, have a lot to gain from channeling their Vulnerable expression. Even though you are comfortable expressing your emotions in a creative way, allowing yourself to soften your tough exterior and be more vulnerable can be difficult. Speaking as a Rebel who knows this all too well, vulnerability is a tough one for me. To be vulnerable, you have to soften, and when you soften, you let your guard down. It's only by letting your guard down and being vulnerable that you can truly allow others to be there for you. This can be hard because in order to let others be there for you, the Rebel Mama has to trust them with her feelings, emotions, and overall being. You spent years of your life building your Rebel walls up to protect yourself from having to depend on others. I look at some of the Vulnerable Mamas I work with and am in such awe. They can be so free and trusting, allowing others to be there for them. It takes a lot of guts and bravery in my book to be that free with one's emotions.

I was at a birth with one of my doula clients who was a Vulnerable Mama. When a lot of fear came up, she reached out to her husband and to me for support, allowing herself to experience raw emotions. The relationship between her and her partner was so beautiful. He was able to be there for her and allowed her to just be. Being vulnerable is the only way to have true intimacy, not only with your partner, but also with other moms. When you can soften and not be so tough all the time, you become more real and allow others to connect with you on a deeper level than ever before.

rebel mama toolkit

Rebel Recipe:
Hibiscus, Cinnamon, and Ginger Tea

You have no problem taking risks and charging forward, but it can feel tough to slow down and recharge. Self-care is necessary if you're going to take on the world, and this warm, spice-tinged tea handcrafted by Heng Ou can help. Hibiscus helps soothe inflammation while cinnamon keeps your fire stoked, supporting libido and fighting depression.

SERVES 4

• *2 cinnamon sticks*

• *1-inch (2.5-cm) knob of fresh ginger, peeled*

• *1/4 cup (10 g) dried hibiscus blossoms*

• *2 tablespoons honey or organic agave nectar*

➤ Bring 4 cups (960 ml) water to a boil in a small pot, along with the cinnamon sticks and fresh ginger. Turn the heat down to low, add the hibiscus blossoms, turn off the heat, cover the pot, and let it steep for 20 minutes.

➤ Strain and sweeten as desired and sip throughout the day.

✳ Rebel Supplements:
Stress Less

Elissa Goodman recommends these nutritional supplements to balance your system and help recharge your body when it needs rest and recovery.

Life Extension Neuro Magnesium: This supplement acts as a calming agent that settles the overthinking mind so you can focus better and make intentional decisions.

Pure Encapsulations B-Complex Plus: This can help balance your emotions so you can handle pressure and not feel rushed.

Gaia Ashwagandha: This herb is known to help reduce the feelings of stress and anxiety.

☀ Rebel Oils:
Soften and Soothe

All these oils can be diffused, added to a bath, or worn as a healing perfume. A lot of essential oil blends often contain hidden chemicals, so I recommend Young Living Essential Oils for their high-grade quality and purity.

YOUNG LIVING ESSENTIAL OILS

Inner Child: to help nurture your child self within

SARA: for emotional release and healing

Gentle Baby: to soothe your spirit

✳ Rebel Crystals:
Embrace New Energy

When you first get your crystal, you have to solidify your bond. As with any relationship, it takes time for your energies to sync. For a crystal to purify your energy, you have to first return the gesture and cleanse its energy. You can let your crystal bathe outside in the light of the sun or moon for at least four hours, or place it on the soil or hang it on the branch of a healthy houseplant for twenty-four hours. Then sit quietly, holding the stone in both your hands. Visualize your intention for the crystal. The stone is listening. Giving your crystal a job allows you to set your intention for the work you'll do together. It's okay to get specific! After programming the crystal with your intention, your crystal is now activated. Heather Askinosie has chosen these crystals specifically to help Rebel Mamas soften and open.

Unakite: When the Rebel Mama feels herself being pulled or pushed in directions that she's not ready to move in, embracing the energy of unakite will help her remain spiritually grounded. This grounding force provides useful insights that allow her to better understand why she is resisting something and what is really causing her to feel conflicted. Unakite is also known for removing negative emotions stored in the heart, which may have the effect of clearing the inaction that can at times plague the Rebel Mama. Holding the unakite stone, she can ask herself, *Am I being rebellious because I am afraid, or is this feeling stemming from somewhere else?* The energy of transformation in unakite demands that you stay present in the moment so that it becomes difficult to stay stuck in patterns or situations that no longer serve you.

Amazonite: This stone's energy reminds you that being in the flow is where the magic of life resides. When the rebellious nature goes from being a strong suit to a weakness that is impeding personal progress, it's beneficial to consult amazonite energy. Amazonite forces you to trust the flow and rebel *against* your naturally rebellious instincts.

Nuummite: Nuummite will help the Rebel Mama embrace the shadow side of her personality, instead of pushing away unwanted or uncomfortable feelings. Empowered by the nuummite energy, the Rebel Mama will take on her darkness with a "bring it" attitude and grow closer to the light as she moves through the dark.

rebel yoga:
cooling the inner fire

This sequence is all about softening the edges and cooling your internal fire. These postures are designed to help soften, open, and relax your mind and body.

Suggested props: mat, bolster, yoga blanket or towel

✳ Breath Work

- Set a timer for 3 minutes. Start in a seated position and close your eyes. Begin to breathe in through your nose for a count of 4 and exhale out your nose for a count of 6—make the exhale slower than the inhale (when the exhale is longer, it cools and grounds). Feel the life force energy, or *prana*, move throughout your body from your head down through your feet, and as you exhale, scan your body from the ground up, softening and relaxing. Notice the sounds, the smells, the air that's all around you, and without opening your eyes, see your surroundings with your intuition. See if you can merge the rhythms of your breath and that of the earth, becoming part of the bigger whole.

✳ Knee Rocks

- Now lie on your back and bring your knees into your chest. Rock to each side for a few seconds. With your knees by your chest, place your hands on the front of the knees. Inhale for 4 counts and exhale for 6 counts, pushing your knees away from your chest and keeping your feet off the floor. Inhale and bring them back up to your chest, and exhale and push away for 6 counts. Repeat this 10 to 12 times, linking your body with your breathing, feeling the support of the earth beneath you.

✳ Half Happy Baby

- Place a bolster vertically to the left of your torso. Bring your right knee in toward your chest and hold, breathing into the tension and exhaling out any hardness in your lower back as your body surrenders deeper into the ground.

- Grab the sole of your right foot with your right hand or make a hook with your pointer finger and middle finger and hook under your big toe. Bring your right knee down to the ground toward your armpit and right foot above. Hold and explore where you can soften the energy. Slowly bring the bent leg back toward your chest and twist it across your body to the left side, resting your knee on the bolster. Turn your head toward your knee and surrender into this restorative twist. Breathe in through your nose for a count of 4 and think of something joyful, then breathe out through your mouth for a count of 6 and think of something that recently pissed you off. Continue breathing in the positive and releasing any negative energy, softening the edges of the ribs as you exhale (if your neck starts to hurt, gently turn it to the other side).

- Bring both knees into the chest, move the bolster to the other side, and switch legs. Bring the left knee in toward your chest and then twist over to the bolster. This time, breathe in gratefulness and exhale out any resentment or bitterness. Hold each side twist for 3 minutes.

✳ Spine Stretch

- Bring both knees back toward your chest and straighten your legs out on the ground as your reach your arms over your head. Stretch your feet as far away from your hands as you can, feeling taller and more energetic. Hug your knees back in toward your chest and roll over to the right side.

✳ Side Stretch

- With your knees tucked underneath you, face the floor and extend your arms out above your head, with your palms resting gently on the floor (child's pose). Breathe in deeply to the back of your heart through your nose and exhale out any judgment or frustration. Crawl both hands over to the right, inhale, and continue breathing with intention as you soften this area of your body. Breathe in and out 3 times, then walk both hands to the left side and repeat. Continue inhaling with compassion, empathy, and love, exhaling misunderstanding, frustration, or impatience with yourself or others.

✳ Cat/Cow

- Now lift your back with your knees on the floor, hip-width apart, and your hands on the floor under your shoulders. Slowly arch your back and look up as you breathe in through your nose, and look down as you exhale through your mouth. Feel yourself breathing in flexibility and breathing out any hardness or stubbornness.

✳ Camel with Cooling Breath

- Come up onto your knees with your toes tucked under your feet, and place your hands in front of your body at the top of your rib cage by your diaphragm. Visualize a big yellow fire. Reach back behind you, grab your heels with your hands, and arch your back. Purse your lips and inhale with your mouth as if you are breathing in through a straw, then exhale through your nose. Imagine you are a fire-breathing dragon. Do this for 3 complete breaths, then sit back on your heels and rest for a few seconds. Repeat 2 more times.

✳ Restorative Twist

- Sit back on your heels and slide your butt over to the left of your mat, keeping your knees bent. Place the bolster perpendicular to your right hip, bring both hands to each side of the bolster, lay your torso and chest flat on the bolster, and turn your head to the left with your right cheek resting on the bolster. You can place your hands to hug the top of bolster. Take slow, deep breaths—there's nothing to do here but surrender to this pose. Breathe VERY slowly and deeply in through your nose, and in your mind (or out loud), think or say the following and allow your body to respond:

(Inhale) *I* (exhale) *surrender*

(Inhale) *I* (exhale) *let go*

(Inhale) *I* (exhale) *relax*

(Inhale) *I* (exhale) *soften*

(Inhale) *I* (exhale) *trust*

(Inhale) *I* (exhale) *flow*

(Inhale) *I* (exhale) *receive*

- After you've completed the phrases (or 3 to 5 minutes of breathing), come up and switch sides. Repeat.

✳ Restorative Chest Opener

- Roll up a yoga blanket or towel and place it horizontally on the ground behind you. Lie back so the blanket is where your bra strap would be. Raise your arms above your head with your elbows bent. Breathe in deeply through your nose into your diaphragm (in between your ribs) and feel that area expand and open. As you exhale through your mouth, soften and surrender deeper into the pose. Think of filling your body with a white or golden light and expelling any darkness. Continue breathing for 3 to 5 minutes.

- Come back to child's pose, and bring your arms alongside your body. Begin to rock gently forward and back or side to side. Come up to a comfortable seated position and take a few minutes to notice how you feel. Did something come up for that you wanted more of or needed to work on? Think of two actions you can take to invite more of this energy.

rebel affirmations:
trust the universe

Take a look at these words and phrases and notice if any jump out at you or give you an "aha!" feeling. If so, consider saying them out loud or taping a handwritten version somewhere so you can read them daily. You could also try adding images to make a vision board.

I SOFTEN.

I AM OPEN.

I EMBRACE MY INNOCENCE.

I AM OPEN TO RECEIVING.

I RECEIVE.

I PUT MYSELF IN OTHERS' SHOES.

I AM COMPASSIONATE AND EMPATHETIC.

I AM OPEN TO WAYS OF BEING OTHER THAN MY WAY.

WHEN PEOPLE GIVE ME ADVICE,
THEY HAVE MY BEST INTEREST AT HEART.

I TRUST.

I LISTEN.

I BEND.

I TAKE PAUSE AND BREATHE
BEFORE REACTING.

rebel meditation:
bend your mind

In balancing strength and vulnerability, think of yourself as a bamboo pole. Bamboo is one of the strongest reeds in nature, yet it is able to bend so it doesn't break. There is much more strength in balance. This meditation from Michele Meiche will create balance between your thinking mind and the feelings in your body.

For this mindful moment, stand with your feet shoulder-width apart. Soften your legs and knees by keeping your knees slightly bent. Your eyes can be open or closed. If your eyes are open, soften your gaze to relax the muscles in your face. If standing is not comfortable for you, this mindful moment can be done sitting or lying down.

Take a relaxed deep breath in and really feel your strength. Pause your breath in a relaxed way and feel your body tall and sturdy like a bamboo pole as you think about the times you have been strong.

As you breathe out, bring your shoulders back and down and let your body soften like a bamboo pole bending in the wind. Feel the flexibility of openness and softness in your body.

Begin to breathe in for a count of 3 and feel your strength in your body and mind. Breathe out for a count of 3 as you feel softness and opening in your body and mind. Repeat this same inhale/exhale 2 more times. Now breathe in for a count of 3 as you feel your strength in your body and mind, and breathe out for a count of 3 as you feel flexibility and opening in your body and mind.

Let your breath return to its own natural rhythmic pattern, all the while feeling your inner strength, openness, and flexibility in your body and mind.

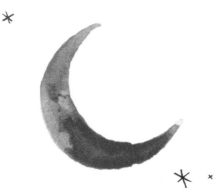

deepening your self-awareness

Answer these questions in order as they build upon each other, to continue understanding and connecting with your inner Rebel Mama expression:

1. Where does or where has your Rebel expression shown up in your life?

2 What do you resist or find most off-putting about Rebel Mamas?

3. Where do you resist this aspect of the Rebel Mama expression within yourself?

4. Who's your favorite Rebel Mama, and what do admire about her?

5. Where can you see parts of her reflected in you?

6. How might your life change from integrating more of your Rebel expression into your life and being?

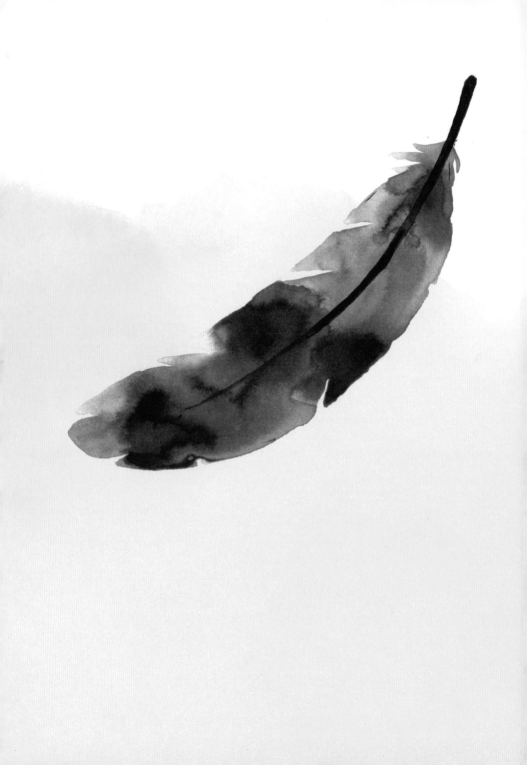

chapter six

VULNERABLE MAMA

Can't Stop the Feeling

~~~~~~~~~~~~~~~~~~~~~~~~

I'm always in awe of women who are able to ask for and receive help with ease, and allow others to be there and care for them. In today's busy, competitive world, many of us pride ourselves on being strong, and we forget that there is an immense power in expressing vulnerability. The Vulnerable Mama harnesses her natural curiosity and openness, seeks out extra attention and support, and wisely uses "the village" to help her raise her family. There is a beautiful innocence about her and her yearning to learn and take direction well.

I probably don't have to remind you that it's hard being a woman these days! There is so much pressure from work stress, family obligations, maintaining a solid relationship, keeping up with the Joneses (on social media and IRL!), and the list goes on and on.

All this pressure can toughen a gal up and push her into channeling more male energy. Oftentimes strength is the only thing women focus on, because it seems you have to be strong just to exist. The good news is that channeling an expression of Vulnerability can allow you to feel more and express your emotions more easily. Vulnerable Mamas might think they feel more afraid or anxious at times than other moms, but I'm gonna let you in on a little secret: all mothers at some point feel fear and anxiety. Most just mask it or deal with it differently. Remember, even if it's not your primary expression, all mamas have different levels of Vulnerability within them.

When I work with Vulnerable Mamas, they respond to my services very well. They reach out; we talk. And then they reach out to their doctor, mother, sister, friend, partner, and even their freakin' dog! They come back to me feeling more confused than ever. The oversaturation of information on the internet as well as the overexposure to what people choose to share on social media doesn't help, either. Our age of technology feeds into fear, breeds insecurity, and can confuse your personal sense of right and wrong, leaving you doubting what you know to be true for you. I can tell you one thing for sure: if you're looking for a problem, you sure as hell will find it on the internet!

If you are nodding your head, this chapter is for you. And I'll help you remove some of that angst and anxiety. One way is to limit your time on social media and stop using Dr. Google. Yes, really, it's that simple. When clients show up expressing Vulnerability, I act as a sounding board, asking them specific questions to quiet the external noise and help them find their truth within. Once they find it, I empower and encourage them to follow it. You'll find exercises and practices to empower yourself to do the same here!

BE PRESENT

Have you noticed that you are always waiting for the other shoe to drop? Or do you find yourself asking questions that start with, "What if, what if, *oh shit, not again,* what if," all day long? Girl, let me tell you: the *what ifs* and *oh shits* are dragging down your quality of life, and that is downright exhausting and no way to live. You may want to take some cues from your Flow Mama friends on this one to help you connect with your inner Flow and be more present. They are amazing at living in the moment and going with whatever way the wind is blowing at the time.

When you are in your Vulnerable expression, often you live in a place of worry, always on guard. One of the main reasons we experience fear is that we are living in the future, which is fantasy, or in the past, holding on to or reliving something that already happened. In either case, you are definitely not in the present. You can let go of so much once you realize this present moment right here and now is all there really is. It's what you do now that creates your tomorrow. The only thing you have control over is how you choose to show up today. When you feel a case of the *what ifs* or the *oh shit, not agains* coming on, the best thing to do is bring yourself to the here and now and focus on what's going on today.

If you can channel your anxiety and worry by turning it into curiosity and wonderment, it will help you thrive. This is almost like what a child does through learning by play. When you learn through play, you figure it out as you go. Getting in touch with your inner Flow helps keep you living in the moment. One of the positive attributes of the Flow Mama is that she goes where she is being pulled to, and therefore, she makes decisions from what's happening in the present moment.

I was practicing fertility yoga and coaching with one of my girls, a Vulnerable Mama with a lot of fear and anxiety. She had been trying to get pregnant for three years. One day, during a session, I guided her through some postures and questions that took her deep within. She discovered that the root of her anxiety was a fear that she would turn into her parents if she had a child. This Vulnerable Mama was living in the past. She and her husband had an amazing relationship, but her relationship with her parents? Well, let's be kind and just say, not so much. I encouraged her to do the Reality Check exercise on page 136.

On two pieces of paper, she wrote the qualities she and her husband had as a couple and the qualities her parents had. Sometimes writing it side by side and seeing it on paper emphasizes the differences and allows for a clear vision of the truth. Because let's face it, when it's in your head, it can just be a jumbled mess.

I asked my client to release her fears by writing about it with the ritual PEW-12 Writing (see page 139). Instead of burning it right away, I asked her to read it to her husband, who said, "OMG, babe, that's so not happening to us! Let's burn that shit!" So they burned it together.

Next I asked them to write vows for their relationship and family, post-baby. They then wrote out steps they could take now that would carry them into their future together After three years of trying, she got pregnant the next month and they now have a beautiful baby boy. And their post-baby relationship and family vows are still hanging in their bathroom, to remind them daily of their intentions.

*DROP IT LIKE IT'S HOT

Vulnerable Mamas *feel* strongly, and in today's world, where so many repress their feelings, this is such a positive quality to be able to embody. But it can get you into trouble when you get swept up in a hurricane of your own feelings and emotions. You react from a place that is not grounded or centered. This is a great time to step away, burn off some of the meshuggaas (y'know, the *cray-cray*), and shift your energy before communicating or making important choices. Again, it's what we do in the present that creates our future. We want to make decisions from a calm, grounded place and our truth, not an emotional or highly charged place.

Play your favorite dance music for 3 to 5 minutes (or as long as you're enjoying yourself!). Close the door, turn it up, and drop it like it's hot. Shake your booty and BURN your worries right off. You are literally moving, clearing, and shifting your energy. It's nearly impossible to worry while you're singing your heart out and dancing freely!

where are you living: past, present, or future?

All of a sudden you are having an out-of-body experience. Something has triggered you, but you're just not sure what. All you know is that you're not feeling great because you are caught up in a worry-storm that's causing you to topple over and lose your ground. Try this:

> STOP yourself the minute you feel that familiar feeling of worry.

> Bring yourself back to the present moment by noticing your surroundings, feeling your feet planted firmly on the ground, and acknowledging today's date.

> Which one of these questions—(a) or (b)—can you answer in this moment? There is a chance that you could be going to the past and the future at the same time (yikes!):

  a. Does something you are worried about feel familiar (i.e. *Oh shit, not again!*) If so, what?

  > Make a list of what is different today versus what happened in that past experience, making note of the big differences and the subtle ones as well.

  > If you are having a hard time letting go of a trigger or an event from the past, skip to page 139 to learn how to do the PEW-12 exercise to help clear this energy.

  > Take note of all the things that are going right in your life.

  > Give gratitude and take a moment to count your blessings for all that you have and are today.

b. Are you thinking about something in the future that may or may not happen? (i.e. *What ifs!*) If so, what?

➤ Ask yourself if there is a real issue happening today. If there is, can you do anything about it? If so, write out what actions you can take today or at this present time to help you step more gracefully into the future. Do them.

➤ If there is nothing to be done now, try the PEW-12 writing on page 139 to help clear and move some of this energy.

➤ Take note of all the things that are going right in your life.

➤ Give gratitude and take a moment to count your blessings for all that you have and are today.

✳ FREE YOURSELF FROM FEAR

Clearing out our emotional closet can be terrifying at first, but once we survive what we didn't think was survivable, we'll get a taste of our limitless power to heal and change.

—DR. HABIB SADEGHI,

FOUNDER OF BE HIVE OF HEALING INTEGRATIVE MEDICAL CENTER

All mamas have some level of fear, but I find it to be especially present with my Vulnerable Mamas. So the question is, what do we do with our fears? I was hanging with one of my fabulous clients, doing a birth prep session along with her husband, working through any fears they had about parenthood or birth. She said, "I'm good, I feel totally relaxed, excited, and free of any blocks or fears." A little surprised, I said, "Wow, that's amazing! How are you doing that?"

She shared with me a daily ritual her teacher, Dr. Habib Sadeghi, taught her called PEW-12 that helps clear the emotional junk that many of us carry. Since that day I have made this part of my morning ritual, and I can't tell you what a huge difference it makes in my energy level and emotional state. It's like taking the trash out daily instead of letting it build up, clutter, and stink up the house. I am so incredibly grateful for this gift she shared with me! I incorporate this ritual with my fertility clients as well as with my moms-to-be, new moms, and their partners.

PEW-12: purge writing ritual

The number 12 symbolizes balance and represents an end and a beginning of a cycle (12 hours in a day, 12 hours in a night, 12 months in a year).

Gather the following materials:

- *1 white candle (The white candle absorbs, protects, and clears your space from toxic and negative energy.)*

- *Matches*

- *A timer*

- *A large pad of paper*

Now follow these steps:

➤ Light your candle.

➤ Set a timer for 12 minutes. (I use the one on my iPhone.)

➤ Write about something that's bothering you or holding you back or any unresolved issues you might have where you haven't been honest with yourself or with others. Let all your emotions go onto the paper and out of your body as you purge your mind, body, and spirit free of any negative energy you might be carrying within. Don't stop until the 12 minutes are up. Wherever you are when the timer goes off, stop writing.

➤ DO NOT READ WHAT YOU WROTE. (You don't want to put it back into your subconsciousness.)

➤ Burn the paper somewhere safe (in a fireplace, sink, barbecue, etc.). Fire changes the chemical composition of things, and therefore burning the paper symbolizes a shifting of energy.

➤ Blow out your candle.

➤ Repeat daily until you begin to feel emotional freedom.

☀ FIND YOUR TRUTH AND BELIEVE IN IT

When working with Vulnerable Mamas, I have noticed that you often don't trust yourselves. You tend to seek advice outside of yourself instead of following your intuition, which causes you to easily get swayed by other people. This adds up to losing your sense of self and truth. The challenge here is that you can't trust yourself unless you know and accept yourself. You've spent a good portion of your life relying on other people to make decisions for you. In other words, you are looking outward instead of inward.

To further hone your intuition, practice the Human Pendulum exercise on page 77 in the Flow Mama chapter. See, you're not the only one who struggles with embracing this incredible gift we all have. All mamas can benefit from strengthening their intuition. It's the perfect antidote for a hell of a lot of challenges!

If you don't trust yourself or the flow of life, you will continue to be thwarted by the fear of constant indecision. Ask yourself, where does your distrust come from? Why don't you trust the universe or yourself? You are one of a kind. What might work for another might not work for you. If you don't understand the way you tick, how can you follow what you know to be true?

One of my clients, Emily, is a dynamic woman, but she doesn't trust herself. Because of this, she looks for outside advice all the time. This impacts her parenting in a big way. Emily called me in the middle of the night crying because her baby was screaming and she was on the fifth day of sleep training. "I can't do this anymore!" she cried. I asked why she was doing this, and she said, "All my friends said this was the right way to get her to go to sleep."

"How does that make you feel?" I asked her. She said that it broke her heart, and that she felt her baby wasn't ready, to which I replied, "I think you have your answer." I helped Emily quiet the noise around her and listen to her inner truth. Her friends were not raising her baby, *she* was. I encouraged her to empower herself to know what was best for her baby and her family.

The latest books, apps, podcasts, and Facebook posts can all make any mama in her Vulnerable expression lose trust in herself. I like to remind my new moms that they can be their own doula in motherhood—try to collect information in a way that informs you to ultimately make your own choices. You and your child are unique, so no advice or program will work unless you tweak it and make it yours. It's fine to take outside advice as long as you're also willing to throw it out if it doesn't work for you. All mamas handle this motherhood doula-ing differently: Action Mamas are queens of information gathering, Flow Mamas are great at staying flexible as they try new things, Free Mamas receive advice objectively, and Rebel Mamas ultimately do their own thing.

Spending too much time looking outside yourself for answers can make you spin out in fear. With trust, the fear will dissipate. Every day we have decisions and choices to make, and your friends or loved ones might not always be available to answer questions or direct you. Some of my best teachers gave me the tools to access my intuition and help me connect to my own sense of what felt right or wrong. This is a skill I can access anywhere, at any time. No cell phone or website can promise you that!

*TRY AN ADVICE DETOX

Set an intention for one week not to ask anyone for their advice. Yes, I'm serious! Think about your need to seek advice as if you're hooked on sugar. *I can't get through the afternoon without cookies.* But in your case, it might be, *I don't know what to do until I talk to Pam.* Calling Pam is your craving.

When the craving hits, pause and breathe through it. The cravings mask the feelings that lie beneath the surface. Notice what comes up for you. Maybe you feel something along the lines of, "What if I make the wrong choice? I don't know what to do. I'm scared."

Go a little deeper to find your self-awareness and the root cause of why you do what you do. In other words, what's underneath the cravings? In this example, the root cause under this craving is self-doubt. Now think about how you can do some inner work using the other expressions to help counteract this craving and heal yourself. Rebel Mamas stand in their conviction; Action Mamas know what they want and go for it; Free Mamas aren't attached to outcome; and Flow Mamas live in the present, making decisions from this place. What expression do you need to pull up within yourself? Remember, you possess all of them, and you can use them at any time! Empower yourself to integrate a new way. Usually after sitting with something long enough, through all the discomfort, and not giving in to those cravings, you will find an answer. When you are constantly looking outside for the answers, you don't give yourself a chance or the space to find what rings true for you. Resist the urge to ask others and see where this takes you. Now pat yourself on the back, because you just took the first step in trusting yourself.

A NOTE ON DETOXING: When I do a juice cleanse, the first few days suck. Withdrawal starts to hit, and I feel awful and tempted to quit. But if I stick with it, I start feeling great in a matter of days (sometimes within twenty-four hours). Being uncomfortable is part of the process, and for it to work, you can't rush the process, or you'll miss the critical steps you need to take along the way. Don't be afraid of discomfort! You have to push through and stay on course, even when you are jonesing for a fix. *The only way out is through.* You gotta feel it to heal it. This is where your willpower comes into play. Try the PEW-12 exercise again (page 139), and don't react by giving in to temptation.

A few tips to help ease your way through the discomfort:

- Take 10 slow, deep breaths.
- Download a meditation from YouTube or do Michele's meditation in this chapter (page 162).
- Go for a walk or a workout.
- Purge write.
- Do the yoga sequence in this chapter (page 155).
- Take a relaxing shower.
- Dance.

build a bubble of peace

One of the first sessions I do with my pregnant and new mom clients is to create a Bubble of Peace they can surround themselves with throughout their pregnancy and motherhood journeys. It's not just the foods you eat or the products you use; it's the energy you emit that you and your baby absorb and simmer in. Quiet the noise around you. Seek counsel within.

By creating this Bubble of Peace, you will set an intention for the way you want to feel during your whole motherhood journey.

1. Get cozy in a position that feels good to you.

2. Close your eyes and begin to see yourself.

3. Begin to imagine a big bubble all around you.

4. Visualize a place where you have felt relaxed and at peace, and fill up your bubble with this environment.

5. Use your senses to take you to that place; feel the sun and air, smell the fireplace or sea, hear the sound of the waves or the leaves moving through the trees, see the colors and everything that surrounds you.

6. Come up with 3 to 5 words that describe how you feel in this bubble. (Example: I feel cozy, peaceful, and grounded.)

7. Use these 3 to 5 words to set your intention for motherhood. You are surrounding yourself with this Bubble of Peace energy.

8. Scan your life in the present moment by asking these questions:

> *Who are the people in your life?*

> *Do they feed your Bubble of Peace energy? If so, bring them into your bubble. If not, move them outside your bubble.*

> *What are your thoughts and habits?*

> *Do they feed your Bubble of Peace energy? If so, bring them into your bubble. If not, move them outside your bubble.*

> *Where and how do you spend your time, and what are the places you frequently visit?*

> *Again, bring in all that feeds and supports you and move out all that doesn't.*

> *Ask yourself if there is anything else you can do to have more of the energy that feeds you in your life and bring it into the bubble.*

9. Cut out photos from magazines or download images off the internet that reflect your vibe. Create a vision board or draw your Bubble of Peace. Hang it up somewhere to remember your intention.

10. Hold on to this Bubble of Peace energy as you go through your day. One way to do this is to revisit it before you hop out of bed in the morning. Or, when anxiety or stress is present, take a few breaths and remember your bubble.

detox from the internet

If you're anything like me, you probably need a twelve-step program for social media. I sadly see way too many women feeling bad, questioning, and doubting themselves and their choices, and comparing themselves to others after spending countless hours staring down at their phones. Ironically, there are actually apps to help get your app addiction under control! Here are just a few I've found:

> Offtime (iOS, Android)

> Moment (iOS)

> Flipd (Android)

> AppDetox (Android)

> Stay on Task (Android)

And by the way, those mom chat rooms . . . Oh HELLO, fear! I went on once to see why my clients were freaking out, and I literally had a panic attack reading the crazy things people were typing.

I know it's way easier said than done to ask you to stay off the internet, so try limiting your time. It's so important to take some of that energy you spend looking outward and bring it inward. When I am pondering a choice or making a big decision, I go for a walk by myself in nature and bring my journal. If I don't get what I'm looking for, I do it again, removing myself from the noise of others and technology. Waiting is sometimes the hardest part, but you have to allow for the space for the answers to drop in, and they will eventually come. Be patient with yourself as you are learning a new way to trust yourself.

✳ THERE'S ALWAYS MORE TO LEARN FROM EACH OTHER

I was hanging out one night with a few moms who were gossiping about a woman they'd all met at back-to-school night. The woman they described clearly seemed like a Vulnerable Mama: a "nervous nelly," they said, who asked too many random, off-the-wall questions. Knowing the Vulnerable expression well, I said, "Listen, she's obviously different from you. Her nervousness is her fear showing up. Did her questions reveal any interesting info? I bet she brought up a few topics everyone was thinking about but were too afraid to ask! Good on her to express her needs and concerns so freely!"

The moms got really quiet as they let this sink in. I took the opportunity to delve deeper. How could we *all* tap into our Vulnerable expression more? My friends started opening up, and pretty soon we were all discussing the benefits of asking for help, showing emotion, and letting go of others' opinions. It was amazing! I even threw out a little challenge for them to befriend the Vulnerable Mama and see if her perceived "weakness" might actually be the thing they needed to integrate into their own lives. And, true story, a year later, I saw an Instagram snap of the three of them hanging out together with their kids. *#mamaste*

✳ SEEK (AND TRUST) YOUR OWN INTUITION

All mothers feel fear and anxiety; it's how they handle it that differs. Vulnerable Mama tends to seek out a gazillion people to find answers, which often leaves her still feeling fearful and unsure. It's a bit like the saying *Too many cooks spoil the broth*. When you ask

natural remedies for vulnerable mamas

MaryRuth Ghiyam created this list of top ten supplements, salts, and essential oils to help alleviate stress, find peace, and calm the nervous system for any mama in her Vulnerable expression.

- *Magnesium Spray:* Apply topically to your wrists or the bottoms of your feet to help relaxation.

- *Magnesium Bath Salts or Epsom Salts:* Put in your bath to help relaxation, and if you want to go even further, add a few drops of essential oils like Roman chamomile, lavender, and rose to the water to help calm and create deeper relaxation in your body and nervous system.

- *MaryRuth Organics Nighttime Multimineral:* Take these to help relax the body and mind and promote good sleep.

- *Chamomile Tea:* Sip a cup of this.

- *Lemon, Ginger, and Peppermint Essential Oils:* Add a drop or two of these to drinking water to help soothe digestive problems.

- *Tangerine, Wild Orange, and Bergamot Essential Oils:* Put in a diffuser to help uplift the spirit.

- *Vitamin B12:* Take this to help calm the nervous system and balance moods.

- *Rescue Remedy:* Take this to calm and provide relief from stress.

- *Kava, Poppy, and Valerian Root:* Take this to help calm and relax your nervous energy. (*Note:* Not to be taken during pregnancy or when breastfeeding.)

- *Root Vegetables:* These are a woman's best friend! Try eating sweet potatoes, carrots, beets, parsnips, and rutabaga. Root vegetables help balance hormones, and they provide glucose to the brain, alleviating anxiety and depression while grounding unstable energy.

one hundred different people for advice, you may get one hundred different answers, leaving you more confused than before you even asked. This is where your intuition comes in. You need to seek your guru from within.

All mamas handle fear and anxiety differently. Rebel Mama might do something creative with her anxiety or continue marching down the path she passionately believes in. Action Mama may intellectualize, research the hell out of her fear, and process it out in her head for days. Flow Mama lives in the present moment, but she might look at the pros and cons and let the wind pull her in either direction. And Free Mama has the uncanny ability to disconnect from her feelings and block anxiety out. Remember, you have all these qualities in you. Seek your guru from within.

Without grounding forces, you can spiral into your own anxieties and fears, and start spinning out of control. The other expressions are critical to help you find balance and self-confidence. Accessing your expression of Action creates structure and provides information to feel safe, while tapping into your inner Rebel encourages going within to find your inner guru and truth. Vulnerable Mamas tends to worry and live in a future of *what ifs*, and integrating more Flow can help bring you back to the present moment. While many women go out of their way to avoid pain, the Vulnerable Mama typically feels *everything*—often her mental and emotional pain can manifest in physical pain and ailments, too. By practicing detachment, she can disconnect from whatever is driving the anxiety.

Using all five of her expressions to build trust and resilience creates a safe environment for the Vulnerable Mama to authentically express her innocence and gives her the strength to do what feels right for herself and her family.

vulnerable mama toolkit

✳ **Vulnerable Recipe:**
Sweet Potato and Ginger Tea

Earthy, grounded sweet potato meets the warming influence of ginger in this tea designed by Heng Ou to soothe and calm. Goji berries add a burst of antioxidants that give uplifting influence, helping you maintain a positive outlook and stable mood.

SERVES 4 OR 5

• *1 cup (130 g) peeled, cubed sweet potato*
• *2 slices fresh ginger*
• *1/4 cup (28.5 g) goji berries*

➤ Bring 6 cups (1440 ml) water to a boil in a medium pot. Add the sweet potato cubes to the boiling water. Lower the heat to a simmer and cook for 30 to 45 minutes, uncovered. In the last 20 minutes, add the fresh ginger and goji berries.

➤ Strain and sip throughout the day or store in the fridge for up to 1 week.

✳ Vulnerable Supplements:
Deep Calm

Elissa Goodman recommends these nutritional supplements
to balance your system and restore your body to a calm,
rested state.

Pure Encapsulations Inositol: This supplement lessens nervous
tension and anxiety and can help prevent panic attacks.

Pure Encapsulations L-Theanine: This helps produce a simulta-
neous calming effect and "alert calmness," or a greater ability to
concentrate on mental tasks.

Gaia Kava: This root is used to improve mood, ease anxiety,
and boost sociability. (*Note:* Not to be taken during pregnancy or
when breastfeeding.)

✳ Vulnerable Oils:
Grounded and Safe

All these oils can be diffused, added to a bath, or worn as a healing perfume. A lot of essential oil blends often contain hidden chemicals, so I recommend Young Living Essential Oils for their high-grade quality and purity.

YOUNG LIVING ESSENTIAL OILS

Sacred Mountain: to promote strength, empowerment, and grounding.

Surrender: to help shake off things that are out of your control that may be causing you worry.

Highest Potential: to inspire, empower, and uplift you to be your best self.

✳ Vulnerable Crystals:
Heart Opening

When you first get your crystal, you have to solidify your bond. As with any relationship, it takes time for your energies to sync. For a crystal to purify your energy, you have to first return the gesture and cleanse its energy. You can let your crystal bathe outside in the light of the sun or moon for at least four hours, or place it on the soil or hang it on the branch of a healthy houseplant for twenty-four hours. Then sit quietly, holding the stone in both your hands. Visualize your intention for the crystals. The stone is listening. Giving your crystal a job allows you to set your intention for the work you'll do together. It's okay to get specific! After programming the crystal with your intention, your crystal is now activated. Heather Askinosie has chosen these crystals specifically to help Vulnerable Mamas find balance.

Rose Quartz: Feeling safe is the highest vibration of love. For the Vulnerable Mama whose openness is her strength as well as her weakness, the protection and assurance of emotional safety that rose quartz radiates is essential.

Botswana Agate: The Vulnerable Mama knows that life has many twists and turns. Being open-hearted makes the ebb and flow of feelings more intense, as they are welcomed in rather than walled off. Botswana agate is a great energetic partner for Vulnerable Mamas to have, because it is a stone of healing and stability. It protects against the spiraling out of anxiety by grounding Vulnerable Mamas in calm, self-healing energy. By tapping into Botswana agate's energy, the Vulnerable Mama can allow negativity to wash past her in a way that does not close her off. After all, her vulnerability is her power as well.

Labradorite: Our village is more than the network of people around us. It also consists of the healing energy offered by the earth. Labradorite opens our hearts to the vast energy that we can tap into to achieve success, spiritual restoration, a sense of wonder, and more. The Vulnerable Mama knows that she can reach out to others when she needs help. Labradorite will remind her that she can reach out to the energy of the earth to infuse her with greater power.

vulnerable yoga:
connect with your power

~~~~~~~~~~~~~~~~~~~~~~~~~~

This sequence was designed to help calm the nerves, relax the body, and ground and activate your power center.

Suggested props: mat, yoga block, bolster

 Pelvic Breathing

- Lie on your back on the ground, feet flat on the floor and hip-width apart with your knees bent and hands out by your sides.

- Inhale as you arch your lower back and breathe in for the count of 4 as if you are breathing in the earth. Keep your tailbone and mid back on the floor. Exhale for 8 counts as you slowly press your spine down into the ground, feeling your spine sink deeper into the earth with every exhale. Do this 10 times.

 Shimmy the Knees and Twist

- Keep your feet flat on floor, knees up (as you did with pelvic breathing). Shimmy your knees over to the right to the floor and then to left to the floor. Keep going back and forth for 6 counts and then hold both knees over to the left.

- Place your left foot on top of your right knee and look over to your right side. Breathe into any tightness in your body. Inhale peace into your kidney area; exhale out any fear. Inhale into the side of your body. Exhale calmly anything that is worrying you. Inhale harmony into your kidney area and exhale anything that's causing you anxiety. Shimmy your legs 6 more times and then repeat the twist on the other side, doing the same intentional breathing.

✳ Supported Bridge with Purge Breathing

- Come back to center where you started, feet on the floor and knees up. Grab a block and place it vertically under your tailbone. If it is too high, turn it sideways. As you inhale, breathe in for 4 slow breaths through your nose into your lower belly and lower back, and as you exhale, breathe out through your open mouth, making a *Haaaaaaa* sound for 4 slow counts. This breath is super powerful for moving and clearing energy.

- Inhale as you fill yourself up with love; exhale any fear.

- Inhale, filling yourself up with happiness; exhale as you let go of any sadness.

- Inhale peace; exhale any stress.

- Inhale faith; exhale any doubt.

- Inhale confidence; exhale any insecurity.

- Inhale clarity; exhale any confusion.

- Inhale trust; exhale any distrust.

- Inhale forgiveness; exhale any anger or resentment.

- Inhale joy; exhale any depression.

- Inhale gratitude; exhale any impatience.

- Inhale light; exhale any darkness.

- Inhale health and vitality; exhale any sickness or toxins.

- Inhale something you need more of; exhale something you need less of.

- Inhale something you are hoping for; exhale any blocks that might be preventing you from having it.
- Inhale the present moment; exhale out the past (it's over and gone).
- Inhale the present moment; exhale the future (you're creating it now).
- Inhale the present moment; exhale this present moment.
- Remove the block and very slowly, one vertebrae at a time, bring your hips to the ground and hug your knees into your chest. Rock side to side.

✳ Reclining Pigeon Pose

- Still lying on your back, put your left foot on the ground and cross your right foot over your left knee. Thread your right hand through the space between your legs, and move your left hand around, grabbing the back of your thigh or above the left knee; hug your knee in toward your chest. Your hips are a dumping ground for emotions. Breathe into the hip area or where you are feeling tension, and as you exhale, let go of any unwanted emotions, negative thoughts, or habits no longer serving you. After a few rounds of this breathing, switch sides and repeat. When you are finished, hug your knees back into your chest, roll over to the right side, and make your way up into a seated position.

✳ Breath of Fire

- This powerful breath helps activate your power center—the third chakra—and strengthen the nervous system.

- Come into a cross-legged seated position. If it would be more comfortable, sit on a bolster. Place both hands over your diaphragm area, between your lower front ribs. Close your eyes.

- Inhale through your nose for no longer than a second and exhale through your nose for the same length of time as you pull your belly button back toward your spine. It's rapid. Keep going for 1 minute. On your last breath, take a deep breath in, hold for 10 counts, and exhale. Wait a few seconds and then repeat the above 2 more times for a whole minute each time.

- Still in the same position with your eyes closed, rest your hands on your knees. Scan your life and notice where you gave your power away because of fear. See all the people and events where you looked outside yourself and allowed others or things to control the way you feel, or think of times when you put your own power in their hands by allowing them to make choices for you. Start to imagine a magnet facing out in front of you in your diaphragm area. Call back all the power you gave away and visualize yellow light pouring back into this area of your body. Notice who or what pops in.

✳ Cross-Legged Forward Bend

- Come into a cross-legged forward bend. Walk your hands out in front of you on the floor and fold forward. Breathe into any tension in your hips; exhale out as you soften and relax this area. Breathe in something you need more of and breathe out any unwanted emotions through your mouth. Remember, the slower and deeper your breath, the calmer you will become. After a few rounds, switch sides, bringing your opposite foot in front, fold forward again, and repeat.

✳ Butterfly Pose

- Put your feet together facing each other and allow your knees to fall out to the sides on the ground. Inhale the length of your spine, exhale, and fold forward. Breathe into any tension as if your breath was magic healing energy. Exhale as your whole body relaxes and softens. Repeat 5 to 10 times.

✳ Legs-out-in-Front-of-You Seated Forward Bend

- Put both legs out in front of you on the floor, reach your arms over your head, exhale, lengthen your spine, and fold forward. Take 5 to 10 slow, deep breaths.

✳ Legs-up-Wall with Bolster

- Bring your bolster and mat over to a wall. Leave about an inch of space between the bolster and the wall. Sit sideways on the bolster and swing your legs up the wall as your torso falls back onto the ground. If you need to adjust yourself, scoot your butt to the center and closer to the wall. Open your legs wide apart on the wall with legs straight (split on wall). Hang out like this for 3 minutes. Slowly walk your feet together and keep your legs straight up the wall for 3 minutes more. Cross your legs at the wall, hold for another minute, then scoot your butt off the bolster. Rest your crossed legs on top of the bolster for 1 minute, then straighten your legs and place the bolster under your knees for your final pose.

✳ Savasana

- Lying on your back, with your legs comfortably resting on the bolster, squeeze your feet and tighten up all the bones and muscles and relax them.
- Tighten your legs as hard as you can and then relax this area.
- Tighten your butt and genitals and unclench them.
- Squeeze your stomach and let it soften.
- Tighten your lower, mid, and upper back and allow them to melt into the earth.
- Tighten up your chest, shoulders, hands, and arms, then allow them all to go limp
- Tighten all the muscles and tendons of your jaw, neck, and face, and then let them all loosen.
- Stay here for at least 3 minutes or as long as you'd like,.
- When you are ready, rise into a comfortable seated position. You may choose to practice the affirmations in the next section, or just sit and be. *Mamaste.*

vulnerable affirmations:
trusted and safe

I AM SAFE.

I TRUST THE PROCESS.

LIFE IS HAPPENING NOW.

I HAVE ALL THE ANSWERS I NEED WITHIN.

I TRUST MYSELF.

FEAR IS AN ILLUSION.

I HOLD THE POWER TO CHOOSE ONE THOUGHT
OVER THE OTHER.

I AM HERE NOW.

THIS PRESENT MOMENT IS ALL THERE REALLY IS.

I TRUST LIFE.

THE UNIVERSE HAS MY BACK.

MY THOUGHTS CREATE AND MANIFEST MY REALITY;
I CHOOSE TO LOOK AT ALL THE THINGS
THAT COULD GO RIGHT INSTEAD OF FOCUSING
ON ALL THAT COULD GO WRONG.

NO NEGATIVE VIBES.

vulnerable meditation:
centered and connected

If you tend to feel more vulnerable, think of yourself as feeling quite a lot. Perhaps you feel that you have to be "on top of it all," that if you let your guard down, the proverbial other shoe is going to drop. Perhaps you are continually asking others for their guidance and reassurance.

When you don't feel safe, your aura becomes porous. This means you are actually too open to other people and outer influences from family, friends, society, the news, and even what is going on around the world. This can be a good thing. However, living from this place wreaks havoc on our adrenals and our physical and emotional body.

The worry, anxiety, and outer focus drain our vital life force energy. The key is to center in oneself and create a rock-solid foundation inside. One way to feel "centered in self" is to have a robust aura and personal space. Very often when we feel vulnerable we feel too open and exposed. We feel our personal space is somehow compromised and our boundaries are not strong enough to be life enhancing. Our personal space is between 12 to 18 inches around us within our aura. Our aura is 6 to 8 feet around us and blends into the ethers, or earth atmosphere. If you think about it, we really aren't comfortable with people we don't know well when they stand in our personal space. We have a tendency to back away from them.

This meditation from Michele Meiche will strengthen your aura and personal space with energetic boundaries, which will help you feel connected to life but not overly vulnerable.

Take a few minutes to do this daily, especially in the morning to start your day. You can do this mindful moment meditation sitting, standing, or lying down. I do my first meditation while I am still in bed to get up and get going. Also, please don't worry about getting the breath count correct; it is more of a guideline and also gives your mind something to do. When you get into the meditative state, you won't be thinking about your breathing.

Close your eyes and focus on your heart-lung area. Repeat the following exercise 3 times:

Breathe in lightly and easily for a count of 6.

Lightly pause your breath for a count of 3.

Breathe all the way out for a count of 6.

Breathe in for a count of 6.

Now, as you lightly and effortlessly pause for a count of 3, picture and imagine a circle of light above your head.

Breathe into this circle of light.

Then breathe out for a count of 6.

Breathe in for a count of 6.

Then as you lightly and effortlessly pause for a count of 3, picture, imagine, sense, see, and feel a circle of light above your head.

Breathe into this circle of light.

Then breathe out for a count of 6.

Breathe in for a count of 6.

Then, as you lightly and effortlessly pause for a count of 3, picture, imagine, sense, see, and feel a circle of light above your head.

Breathe into this circle of light.

Now, as you breathe out, picture, imagine, sense, see, and feel this circle of light encircling and enfolding you.

Now breathe in your own natural rhythm and pace as you breathe into this circle of light.

As you breathe out in your own natural rhythm and pace, picture, imagine, sense, see, and feel this circle of light encircling and enfolding you.

Bring your inner gaze into your heart-lung area as you focus on each in breath and out breath, feeling more calm, centered, and focused inside.

As you breathe in your own natural rhythm and pace, allow your focus to remain inside right there in your heart-lung area.

When you feel ready, open your eyes, feeling calm, centered, and peaceful inside.

deepening your self-awareness

Answer these questions in order as they build upon each other, to continue understanding and connecting with your inner Vulnerable Mama expression:

1. Where does or where has your Vulnerable expression shown up in your life?

2. What do you resist or find most off-putting about Vulnerable Mamas?

3. Where do you resist this aspect of the Vulnerable Mama within yourself?

4. Who's your favorite Vulnerable Mama and what do admire about her?

5. Where can you see parts of her reflected in you?

6. How might your life change from integrating more of your Vulnerable expression into your life and being?

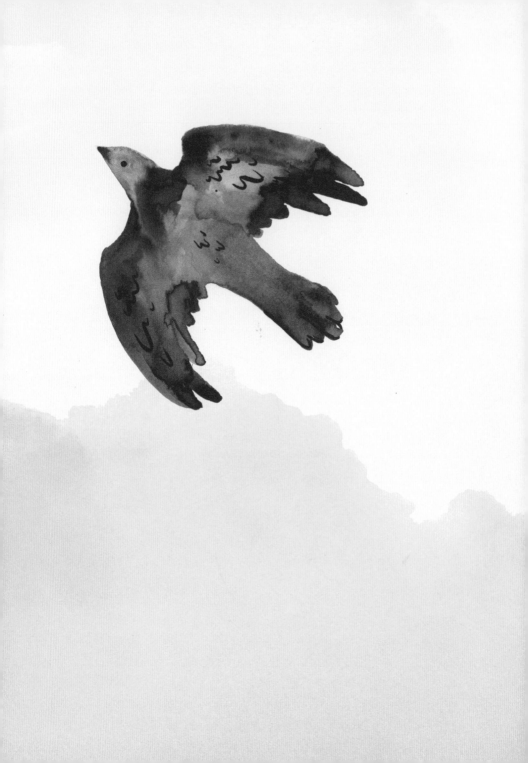

chapter seven

FREE MAMA

Let It Go

~~~~~~~~~~~~~~~~~~~~~~~~~~~~~

I can usually spot a Free Mama at the playground right away—you're the one sitting on a bench, absorbed in a thick, juicy novel and totally lost in your own world while your kids run around enjoying themselves. You let your kids play freely, even if they fall down—because that's what kids do! You trust that they'll pick themselves up, dust themselves off, and get right back in the game. Because you aren't super attached to outcomes, you have the unique ability to approach tasks and opportunities without fear of the future.

But your seemingly free-flowing nature isn't all rooted in trust or freedom. Free Mamas are typically *very* highly sensitive people, and feeling too much can be overwhelming and scary—instead, you may prefer to mitigate the onslaught of emotions by skimming the surface of life instead of diving in too deep. Free Mamas often have unresolved trauma, and a common strategy for dealing with difficulties is to avoid, numb out, or do whatever it takes to keep things easy and light. Living in your own glorious world can sometimes seem like fantasy to others, and you may feel criticized by others who think you need a reality check.

The Buddhists say that the root of all heartache lies in expectations, and motherhood is guaranteed to stir up a Free Mama's pot. When I work with clients who express themselves as Free Mamas, I keep it light. When things get too heavy or real, it can be too much for the Free Mama to handle. Often, her unique sensitivity is at the core of this response—the world is simply too overwhelming for her to live in at times. It can be challenging for other mamas to understand this, but trust me, it's a very real and valid feeling—show me a mom who hasn't grabbed a glass of wine or a pint of Ben & Jerry's after an especially challenging day! I'm sure there were times when things felt so difficult you fantasized about changing the past or making a more promising future. This is simply you expressing your inner Free Mama.

Free Mamas are sometimes misunderstood because they can come off as superficial or having too little depth. I once worked with a Free Mama who, as shit started to get real during the beginning of her labor, started talking about the super-soft pajamas she bought to wear postpartum! Her conversation topic wasn't silly; it was her coping mechanism. When things get too overwhelming for a highly sensitive person, keeping it light is the way they make life a little easier for themselves.

All mamas can take a cue from Free Mamas by just chilling out and flipping through a *People* magazine to lighten the load and step away from the insanity of everyday life. We don't like to admit it, but most of us tend to take life WAY too seriously. How often do you give yourself permission to Netflix and chill? (Okay, maybe just Netflix?) It's never a bad idea to tap into your Free Mama and detach from your life for a bit to lighten the load. It's especially helpful for Action Mamas to practice detachment when perfectionism comes into play, or to tame the inner control freak.

Other expressions can also benefit from practicing some detachment, especially those who lean toward perfectionism or the outcome of goals like Action and Rebel Mamas. For Vulnerable Mamas who get swept up in their own feelings and emotions, detachment can help calm the noise and shut down the spin cycle. And Flow Mamas can practice detaching from the need to people-please. Remember, we all have an inner Free Mama within us, and it's important to be able to unplug from worrying about outcomes or what others think.

There is a huge mindfulness movement happening right now with being present. With technology on the rise and people on the go nonstop, many of us have become more disconnected from ourselves, our reality, and our own lives. This chapter is for any mama finding herself in this expression or with the need to practice nonattachment.

*OVERPLANNING KILLS THE MAGIC

Many spiritually minded people (not just Buddhists) practice nonattachment as part of their mindfulness. In his book *The Seven Spiritual Laws of Success*, Deepak Chopra writes about the sixth spiritual law of success as the Law of Detachment. In order to acquire anything in the universe, you first need to relinquish your attachment to it. This doesn't mean we give up the intention to create our desire, but we give up our attachment to the outcome. Free Mamas are naturally good at this, and all mamas can benefit from integrating a little more detachment into their lives. How often do you project your way or views onto others, especially other mothers? What if you channeled your inner Free Mama by allowing those around you the freedom to exist just as they are? It takes up too much energy to constantly judge others or impose our views of how we think things should be.

To be too attached to things or outcomes can actually mean to be power*less. Think of it this way: you give your power over to what you are attached to.* If you look outside of yourself to find happiness or fulfillment, you're giving your power away and putting it in someone (or something) else's hands. Is a new house or a fancier wardrobe truly going to bring you happiness? Maybe, in the beginning. What if the clothes get damaged? What if the house burns down? The loss of this attachment would affect you but not permanently dictate your power to be fulfilled. When you can practice detaching, whatever you detach from has no power over you.

When you embrace your ability to let go of your attachments, you'll focus more on your own authentic path as a mother, friend, partner, daughter, sister, and so on. You'll stay true to yourself and follow your own instincts and feelings. You'll be able to flow more easily from one expression to another in order to handle whatever is in front of you.

It's motivating to set specific goals and intentions (right, Action Mamas?), but if you can detach even just a little bit from the outcome, you won't find yourself stuck pursuing only one very limited path. One of my favorite quotes from bestselling author Danielle LaPorte is, "Overplanning kills the magic." Tapping into an expression of Free will allow you to enjoy the element of surprise. Something much different from what you expected comes along, and it could be better and more fulfilling than you ever hoped for.

✳ ALLOW THINGS TO UNFOLD

Crystal identified strongly with her Action Mama expression before having children. She had big plans for herself and her future family. During her first pregnancy, in her first trimester, she called me to ask about the best academic preschools. I asked, "What if your child isn't academic? What if he or she is more creative or athletic?" Crystal didn't want to acknowledge the possibility that her child would or could be any other way and quickly changed the subject. When her daughter was born, she was already enrolled in a highly academic preschool. The wheels were in motion for Crystal's plan to be executed.

We lost touch after that but ran into each other about nine years later at a local restaurant. Crystal told me her daughter was creative but really struggled in school. Her self-esteem and confidence had plummeted because she couldn't keep up. Crystal was concerned but still struggled with the decision to change schools to find a more progressive style of education that better supported her daughter's creativity. She still felt attached to the original vision she had for her child, and the more attached she felt, the more they both suffered. Crystal wasn't able to tap into her inner Free Mama, but you can—the ability to detach can be hugely beneficial to you and your family.

✳ARE YOU READY TO BLOOM?

And the day came when the risk to remain tight in a bud was more painful than the risk it took to blossom.

—ANAÏS NIN, AUTHOR AND DIARIST

Free Mamas play it safe when they skim the surface and avoid getting hurt, but that distance can also make it tough to feel fulfilled. Are you missing out from connecting deeply with others and within yourself? How about your intuition? You have to feel it to access it. I understand not wanting to risk getting hurt. But is all this freedom from feelings really serving you? How can you be emotionally available and present for your partner or child if you aren't emotionally available or present with yourself?

Sienna kept things simple and surface-level before she became a mom. When her son, Charlie, was born, it rocked her world. He had a passionate little spirit from day one, and his depth of personality and emotion was a reality check she couldn't avoid. She had a hard time dealing with his wide range of emotions because she had avoided her own for so long. All her years of living "freely" meant she no longer had a grasp on what was "normal" and thought there might be something wrong with her son.

One day, at her neighbor Angel's house for a playdate, Sienna watched Angel's son have an emotional outburst just like Charlie's. Sienna watched in awe as Angel spoke to her son with genuine compassion. Sienna asked, "How did you know what to say to him or what he needed?"

Angel said, "I put myself in his shoes and imagined what it felt like to be sad, disappointed, and frustrated. Then I spoke to him from that place."

You cannot lead anyone further than you have gone yourself. It's hard to have compassion if you haven't experienced or allowed yourself to feel something like it before. By allowing herself to blossom emotionally and be more emotionally available for herself, Sienna could be more present and available for Charlie's needs.

*LOSE YOURSELF WITHOUT GETTING LOST

Let's face it: we *all* have checked out at one time or another when we're supposed to be focused on the task at hand—and more often than not, these days, it's online. I've spent way too much time scrolling through social media than I'd like to admit! Daily life can be difficult or frustrating or boring for all of us, and daydreaming or fantasizing can help us get through rough times. But we often feel guilty for wasting time. How can you enjoy a little freedom from reality without completely flying away?

Laura, primarily an Action Mama, is a successful executive and mom of an energetic toddler. Her weekly schedule is packed, managing a busy office, not to mention coordinating daycare drop-off and pickup with her husband and trying to make the most of their evenings together. Because she's so capable, most weeks fly by without a second thought, but every once in a while, Laura feels the stress of it all back up on her.

When this happens, she uses a little trick her own mom taught her when she was young and feeling overwhelmed with school-work: she takes a "Mental Health Day." She calls in sick and spends

an emotional peel

For Free Mamas, it's best to gently peel back emotions like layers of an onion instead of slicing it right open to the core. Free Mamas have lots of untapped emotions that may have been dormant for years. Remember, we all have an expression of Free Mama within us, so this exercise can also help anyone who needs to get to the root of an emotion and help move the energy. This exercise will allow you to gently become more conscious and present in a whole new way.

> Remove distractions: Create a sacred space. Turn off your electronics. Find a time and space where you can drop in without interruption.

> Get still: Lie down or sit comfortably. Be sure that you're in a relaxed position and not overly tense.

> Breathe slowly and deeply: This will connect your mind and body. Breathe into all parts of your body starting with your feet, scan the front of your body all the way to the top of your head, and go down the back of your body to your feet. Notice where you might be gripping, holding in tension or pain, or any unevenness.

> Name, feel, or see the sensations in your body: Breathe into any sensations that you start to feel and stay with it; if your mind begins to wander, bring it back to the feeling. You might notice that you have tension in your throat that feels like a hand choking you, or a heaviness in your chest as if you were trapped underneath something heavy.

> Massage it out with your breath: See if you can work out any negative sensation by breathing into it and softening and opening that area of your body. Perhaps you can imagine the hand removing itself from your neck and your throat relaxing. Or the heavy thing floating away, allowing your chest and heart to open and soften.

> Ask your body using your intuition (don't overthink it): What feeling or emotion am I holding in here? Just flow with whatever comes up. If you think, *I want to scream with anger when the hand is removed from my throat*, go with it. This allows your body to talk back to you.

> Where is this emotion or feeling showing up elsewhere in your life? Scan your recent history, maybe even the past twenty-four hours. Where or how else has this sensation of anger appeared? At work? At home or with a particular friend? Your mind will want to take you out of this uncomfortable place. It will wander and want to think about something else. Bring it back to the physical sensation and stay with the emotion you are experiencing. I promise you won't be here long. Try to stay for at least 2 minutes and allow your emotions to exist without judging them

> What do I need? Ask the anger why it's there. What does it want? If nothing comes right away, be gentle with yourself. The answer may appear later or when you least expect it, such as in a dream. Once you identify the problem—*My husband never helps me with bedtime*—think about a solution. Is there something you can do to positively help yourself with this feeling?

> Make an intention to take action: What steps or tangible things can you do this week to help understand how to work through the anger to shift this emotion?

> Reward yourself for the effort: Being emotionally balanced and available is hard work. Allow yourself to do something nurturing and soothing for yourself, like taking a yummy bath or curling up on the couch with a hot mug of tea and a cozy blanket.

the day doing something totally luxurious and relaxing, such as reading in bed, shopping online, or catching up on shows her husband never wants to watch. By living in her own little world and pretending she's free of all obligations, even for a couple of hours, Laura recharges herself and is able to plug back into her life with renewed energy and heart.

While it's important to let yourself get "lost" a little, it's also crucial to remain tethered to reality. Many moms I know have experienced a shocking moment when their phone obsession rears its ugly head. My client Jennifer once told me, "My son was only eighteen months old when he grabbed my phone and ran away. He knew it was the only thing that would get my attention!" She and many moms work hard to stay in the moment around their kids. Practice walking the bridge between reality and fantasy so you can access it when you need to, but stay grounded.

✳ FEEL IT TO HEAL IT

One of Free Mama's survival skills is finding a solution or forcing yourself to focus on the positive. It may seem like a helpful tactic, but too often it's a way to further avoid feeling emotions. This was something I myself had mastered. For example, when you feel sad, you tell yourself, *I have so much to be grateful for! I need to count my blessings and focus on all the positive.* Yes, gratitude is wonderful and something we should all practice more of, but for a Free Mama, it can be a diversion from feeling sad. It's important to allow yourself some time to actually *feel* what you are feeling before using the tools to help you move out of the experience. If you don't allow yourself this time and space, you'll miss a crucial step and give these emotions the opportunity to linger and build under the surface. This is where you need to call in the other expressions. It's important to feel it to heal it. You can only sweep the dirt under the carpet for so long before the dirt grows into a mountain!

Channeling an expression of Action can help the Free Mama tap into her inner emotions by creating a structure in which to explore this area—taking things one step at a time can help make them feel less scary. Expressing Vulnerability is risky but rewarding, as it encourages a Free Mama to rediscover true intimacy with herself, her partner, and her children. It's hard to be emotionally available to others if you aren't comfortable being emotionally available to yourself. True intimacy lies just below the surface. Once you can break through some of your protective barriers, you'll find deeper joy and connection in your motherhood experience as well as all the other relationships in your life. By incorporating more Flow, Free Mamas can allow themselves to live more in the moment and "feel" what's right at the time. And incorporating more Rebel energy can give you the courage to go out on a limb and take a risk. It may seem daunting, but think about the last time you truly felt a deep passion for something (or someone)? I know it's easier said than done, but too often we miss out on the rewards because we're too afraid of the risks. Fortune favors the brave!

You are the queen of not being attached to outcome. But when you reconnect with your body and ground yourself with even a little bit of reality, you'll be able to delve beneath the surface and reconnect with your feelings. Use your natural skill of detachment and allow your emotions to flow. Remind yourself that any discomfort is temporary—the one thing you can count on is change.

acupressure for the emotions

So often we think, "If I could just ____, then I'd be happy." I call this the "Last Five Pounds" phenomenon. Whether it's losing the last five pounds, getting the new job, or moving to a bigger house, it's never the thing itself that will bring us happiness. What we're really searching for is a *feeling*. A feeling that all is well. A feeling of being soothed and content. The best part is that we can feel that way no matter what the rest of our life looks like.

I always say that tapping is like acupressure for the emotions. It's so powerful because it goes beyond mind-body therapy. Tapping is a comprehensive tool to rewire our brain. We give a voice to our negative emotions while tapping on meridian points—incorporating the thinking brain, the emotional brain, and the reactive brain (the body). And when you're tapping along with someone else or into a mirror, the mirror neuron systems are integrated, helping us feel as if we're not alone in dealing with the issue, which is an underacknowledged and necessary component of soothing and of health. Whenever your happiness has been hijacked by something external, reconnect with your own emotional happiness using this unique method from Lena George.

Sit in front of a mirror so you can look into your eyes as much as possible while tapping. For a few breaths, close your eyes and simply notice what you notice inside. Then name the emotion you're feeling. Take your time. Open your eyes whenever you're ready, and we'll start tapping. You don't have to tap too hard; keep it a comfortable pressure. Tap in rhythm to how you are speaking the words.

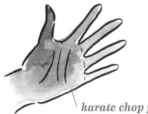

karate chop point

While tapping on the karate chop point:

➤ Repeat 3 times out loud: *Even though I sometimes feel [name the negative emotion or unwanted feeling], I deeply and completely love and accept myself.*

➤ Tap on these 10 points, repeating each statement out loud:
- **Eyebrow:** *Sometimes I get overwhelmed.*
- **Side of Eye:** *Sometimes it feels really hard.*
- **Under Eye:** *Sometimes it feels as if it's all up to me.*
- **Under Nose:** *But maybe my negative feelings are here to help me,*
- **Chin:** *Here to encourage me to practice self-care.*
- **Collarbone:** *Maybe my negative feelings are just what I need,*
- **Underarm:** *Even though they feel bad.*
- **Liver:** *Maybe that's to encourage me.*
- **Wrists:** *To find what I've been looking for.*
- **Crown:** *To let myself receive what I need.*

➤ Take 3 deep breaths and notice what feels different.

Tapping on your own: You can say anything and everything you want while you're tapping. You're never "tapping in negative affirmations"; you're soothing the unwanted feelings, which helps you come out of the threat response. With positive statements you're savoring the wanted feelings, helping the brain register and record the good. Whatever comes up or comes to mind, know that the tapping is giving it just what it needs to restore your well-being.

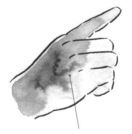

gamut point

The Gamut Point: Notice the indentation on the front of your hand between your ring finger and your pinky finger, just below your knuckles? This is called the Gamut Point. Press on this point during an inhale. On your exhale, release the pressure while making the sound *ahhhhhh*. Repeat 3 times. You can use this little pressure point anywhere, anytime you need a touch of soothing.

Lena recorded this script for you along with a few extras, so follow along with the video if that's easier for you! You can find the video at www.lena-george.com/loribregman.

free mama toolkit

✳ Free Recipe:
Reishi and Shiitake Broth

Sipping a nourishing broth can click you back into your true self. Powerful adaptogen reishi treats anxiety, and shiitake supports energy, helping beat back apathy and emotional paralysis and support energy and courage.

SERVES 6

- *1 white or yellow onion, peeled and roughly chopped*
- *2 leeks, green parts discarded, white parts roughly chopped into coin shapes*
- *2 tablespoons olive oil or a cooking oil such as avocado, coconut, or animal fat*
- *Sea salt*
- *2 cups (70 g) shiitake mushrooms, fresh if possible, or 1 cup (36 g) dried*
- *1 cup (70 g) cremini or white button mushrooms*
- *2 strips kombu (edible kelp/seaweed)*
- *1/2 cup (18 g) dried reishi mushrooms*
- *2 medium carrots, peeled, roughly chopped*
- *1-inch (2.5-cm) knob fresh turmeric, halved*
- *8 cups (2 L) water*
- *1 loosely packed cup (50 g) roughly chopped parsley*
- *2 tablespoons lemon zest*
- *1/2 cup (6 g) fresh dill*

➤ In a medium pot over medium heat, brown the onions and leeks in the oil with a pinch of sea salt.

➤ Run the shiitake, cremini (or white button mushrooms), and the kombu under running water for a quick rinse. Add the mushrooms, kombu, carrots, and turmeric to the pot, along with 8 cups (2 L) water, or enough to cover the veggies by at least 1 inch (2.5 cm).

➤ Cook for 1 1/2 hours over medium-low heat, covered. During the last 20 minutes, add the parsley, lemon zest, and dill.

➤ After cooking, season the broth with salt to taste. Remove from the heat and strain.

➤ Store leftovers in the fridge for up to 5 days, or freeze in zip-tight plastic bags or glass mason jars for up to 3 months.

✳ Free Supplements:
Relax and Calm

Elissa Goodman recommends these nutritional supplements to support your system and help you stay calm and grounded.

Nature's Answer Lemon Balm: This supplement calms down central nervous system damage and supports healing from past trauma.

Thorne PharmaGABA: This supports neurotransmitters, calms the central nervous system, and supports healing from past trauma.

Global Healing B$_{12}$ is needed for neurotransmitter signaling to give you the energy to go about your day without feeling tired and run-down, and at the same time keep your central nervous system calm.

Methylcobalamin B$_{12}$ is the most pure, active, bioavailable coenzyme form of B$_{12}$, and when paired with adenosylcobalamin, the other coenzyme form of B$_{12}$, forms the most potent B$_{12}$ combination available.

✳ Free Mama Oils:
Find Your Fire

A lot of essential oil blends often contain hidden chemicals, so I recommend Young Living Essential Oils for their high-grade quality and purity.

YOUNG LIVING ESSENTIAL OILS

Grounding Oil: to help you feel rooted to the earth

Present Time Oil: to help keep you living in the moment

Transformation Oil: to help ease growing pains and change

✳ Free Crystals:
Get Rooted and Grow

When you first get your crystal, you have to solidify your bond. As with any relationship, it takes time for your energies to sync. For a crystal to purify your energy, you have to first return the gesture, and cleanse its energy. You can let your crystal bathe outside in the light of the sun or moon for at least four hours, or place it on the soil or hang it on the branch of a healthy house-plant for twenty-four hours. Then sit quietly, holding the stone in both your hands. Visualize your intention for the crystal. The stone is listening. Giving your crystal a job allows you to set your intention for the work you'll do together. It's okay to get specific! After programming the crystal with your intention, your crystal is now activated. Heather Askinosie has chosen these crystals specifically to help Free Mamas soften and open.

Smoky Quartz: This crystal helps the Free Mama sink her roots in the energy of Mother Earth. Knowing she is fully supported by this energy helps the Free Mama know that she is free to stand on her own two feet. Being truly free comes from having self-respect and self-love and understanding your personal truth. Smoky quartz is believed to enhance all these aspects of spiritual freedom. As smoky quartz helps the Free Mama respect her strength and get out of her own way, she'll feel less affected by the stress of current and potential problems. This allows the Free Mama to form a foundation for her future, instead of ignoring it to avoid stress in the present.

Tourmalinated Quartz: Keep what works and let go of what no longer serves you, with the energy of tourmalinated quartz. This stone will help the Free Mama focus on the positive and allow that energy to expand and grow. Working with this crystal will increase your ability to release the need to keep moving and plowing forward. Through still reflection with tourmalinated quartz, the Free Mama may come to recognize that the strategy of plowing forward was actually holding her in the same spot.

Leopard Skin Jasper: Similar to a snake that sheds the skin that has run its course, leopard skin jasper energy will bring the Free Mama to shift out of behaviors or mind-sets that she has out-grown. The Free Mama knows intuitively when it is time to move on. When she senses that her tendency to forge through and ignore issues has become counterproductive, the Free Mama can use leopard skin jasper to invoke change in her thoughts, actions, and mind-set. Through this work, she can take on a new, more positive state of being.

free yoga:
creates a strong foundation

~~~~~~~~~~~~~~~~~~~~~~~~~~~~~~~~~

Free Mamas must balance their ability to tune out with a strong sense of their own bodies and feelings, or they run the risk of numbing out completely. I created this yoga sequence to help Free Mamas get back into their bodies and get grounded with the earth.

Suggested props: mat, tennis ball (or small hard ball), bolster, yoga blocks

✳ Grounding Cord

- With your eyes closed, sit in a cross-legged position with your spine straight. Rock forward and back and side to side on your sitz bone (tailbone) and see if you can find a balanced place. Take a few moments to feel and notice your sitz bone on the ground and feel your energy sinking into the earth a bit, as if the ground was giving way. Imagine your tailbone is like a tree trunk going down from this area of your body, deep into the center of the earth. When you get to the center, anchor it here with roots that help ground your energy. (This is something you can do anytime you feel out of your body. It's also a great way to ground yourself before you start your day.)

✳ Opening the Chakras in Your Feet

- Now come up to a standing position and place a tennis ball underneath the middle of the bottom of your foot. Inhale and gently push into the ball, leaning your weight into your foot, and hold. As you inhale, breathe down into your foot; as you exhale, imagine your foot softening like butter as it melts around the ball. Hold here for a few breaths, and then with your eyes closed, roll your foot slowly over the ball in a circle. If you feel tension or tightness, hold it, inhale, exhale, place your weight on it, and massage it out with the ball. When you are ready, switch sides, starting again with the center of your foot, then massaging all around the bottom of your foot.

✳ Find Your Balance

- Put the ball away. Close your eyes and stand with your feet firmly on the ground. Notice how your feet are the foundation that is supporting you. Once again imagine a tree trunk going down into the earth from your tailbone. This time make it thicker, going down into the earth even deeper, expanding out those roots even further.

- Now march in place for 1 minute—march hard, stomping your feet very firmly on the ground. This helps awaken your foot chakras and ground you even more.

✳ Forward Bend

- Stand with your feet hip-width apart, fold forward with a tiny bend in your knees, clasping your hands at your elbows. Sway your torso side to side for a few seconds and then come to stillness in the center; unclasp your arms and place the palms of your hands flat on the ground or up on blocks. Inhale through your nose for 4 counts as you slowly bend your legs. Hold here for 2 counts and exhale through your nose and straighten your legs. Pause for 2 counts and then inhale and bend again for 4 counts, holding the pose and breathing for 2 exhales. Straighten, pausing for 2 seconds before taking your next breath. Keep this going for 10 rounds.

✳ Deep Squat

- Take your feet wider than hip-width apart and turn your toes out to the sides. Bend your knees and come down into a deep squat. Place the palms of your hands together in a prayer position and use your elbows to help pry your knees further apart. Imagine a red balloon on the floor underneath you and breathe it into your perineum area, and as you exhale visualize sending it back down to the ground as you soften, relax, and unclench your butt and genital area. Do this 3 to 5 times.

- From there make your way onto the ground, lying on your back with legs straight and arms at your sides.

✳ Bridge

- Bend your knees, placing the soles of your feet flat on the ground with the palms of your hands flat on the floor at the sides of your body. Inhale through your nose for 4 counts as you lift your hips up and your arms overhead. Pause and hold your breath up at the top for 2 counts and exhale as your arms and hips lower to the ground. Pause for 2 counts before inhaling and raising your arms and hips up, pausing and holding your breath at the top, then exhaling everything. Lower down and pause for 2 counts before the next round. Do this 10 times and then hug your knees into your chest and rock side to side.

✳ Feet-on-Wall

- Lie on your back with your feet hip-width apart on the wall, knees bent in toward your chest, thighs perpendicular to the wall, and hands resting along the sides of your body. Push through your legs into your feet, hold for 30 seconds, and release. Repeat this 3 to 5 times. It's normal for your legs to shake! You are just releasing and moving energy from this area of your body.

✳ Spinal Twist

- With your legs up and knees still bent, bring both legs over to the left and take your arms out to your sides, looking over to the right. Breathe into any tight areas, and as you exhale, allow your body to melt into the ground. Stay here for a few breaths and switch sides.

✳ Spinal Rock

- Hug your knees into your chest and massage your spine by rocking forward and back a few times; then come up to a seated position.

✳ Child's Pose

- Place a bolster or large sofa pillow in front of you and come into a supported pose, where your knees are farther apart than your hips and the bolster is supporting your torso. Your arms are hugging the bolster and your head is turned to the side. Start to rock forward and back like a baby who's self-soothing. Rock for 1 to 3 minutes and begin to ask yourself silently, *What do I need?* Notice if any feeling, words, or visions come up. Now imagine having these needs met. What does that look like?

- Come up into a cross-legged position with your hands in prayer and think of three things you can do to support what you need. *Mamaste.*

free mama affirmations:
honor your emotions

~~~~~~~~~~~~~~~~~~~~~~

Practice saying one or more of these phrases that resonate with you by speaking them to yourself in a mirror once a day, or write them down and stick them somewhere you'll see them daily. You may not feel comfortable at first, but over time, by repeating these affirmations out loud, or writing them out over and over, you'll feel grounded and allow yourself the courage to connect with your body, mind, and emotions.

I CLOSE MY EYES
AND FOCUS ON MY BREATH.
I FEEL MY FEET ON THE GROUND.
THIS WORLD IS A SAFE PLACE TO BE.
I'M ALLOWED TO HAVE FEELINGS.
I'M CONNECTED TO THE WORLD AROUND ME.
I AM HERE NOW.
I FEEL MY EMOTIONS.
I FEEL MY BODY.
I ALLOW MYSELF TO FEEL.

free meditation:
engage with your inner self

~~~~~~~~~~~~~~~~~~~~~~~~~~

Sometimes we feel so much and are overwhelmed, so we don't want to feel more. Many times this "not wanting to feel so much" keeps us from connecting fully to our body as well as to our relationships. When we keep our connection to ourselves and our interactions with others on the surface only, we don't get to our deeper needs, wants, and feelings.

We sometimes skim the surface of our interactions with others and keep things light. We want to see only the positive. In seeing only the light we miss the shadows, hues, and tones of gray of our life. There is a lot to be understood, gained, and felt by going into the full spectrum of life. Part of the depth of our being is in our body. Moving our awareness from our mind to our body gives us a deeper connection to our inner self.

This meditation from Michele Meiche will help you access this depth of connection, inner knowing, and feeling. You will begin to feel this depth of connection within your body and be able to observe it with your mind. This meditation will allow the lightness of your being to blend and harmonize with the depth of your being, as well as bring in more body connection.

Take some time just for you where you won't be disturbed. You can start with 10 to 15 minutes per day. After you have done this meditation for a couple of weeks, you can do 3 to 10 minutes to reinforce your inner connection.

You can also use this meditation anytime you feel scattered, overwhelmed, or disconnected—this will bring you back into body-mind alignment.

Sit in a comfortable, relaxed position, either cross-legged on the floor or seated in a chair with your feet touching the floor and your spinal column in an upright position. Make sure your head is aligned to your spine and not tilting forward or backward.

Close your eyes. Take a deep breath in, and as you breathe in, raise your shoulders toward your ears. As you breathe out, bring your shoulders back down.

Breathe in and bring your shoulders up toward your ears. Breathe out and bring your shoulders backward and downward. Repeat this 2 more times.

Keeping your eyes closed, allow your shoulders to settle into a comfortable relaxed position. Allow your breath to go to its own rhythmic motion as you focus on each in breath and out breath inside. Bring your inner gaze to the bottom half of your body and the soles of your feet. Focus your attention and awareness on the soles of your feet and notice how you feel.

Now bring your inner gaze to the heart-lung area of your body. As you breathe in and breathe out, notice how you feel. Now bring your attention and focus to the top of your head. As you breathe in and breathe out, notice how you feel.

As you take the next breath in, breathing into the top of your head, pause and feel the energy there. As you breathe out, picture, imagine, sense, see, and feel your breath going all the way down the middle of your body to the soles of your feet. Notice how you feel.

Breathe from the soles of your feet back to the top of your head. Notice how you feel.

With your next breath, bring your attention and focus to the heart-lung area of your body. Let your inner gaze focus on your in breath and out breath. Notice how you feel.

Breathe in and out in your natural pace and pattern and notice how calm and centered you feel.

When you are ready you can recite in your mind:

I am calm and centered in my body-mind.

I am comfortable with the lightness and depth of my being.

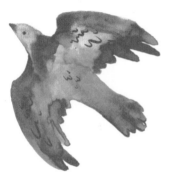

deepening your self-awareness

Answer these questions in order, as they build upon each other, to continue understanding and connecting with your inner Free Mama expression:

1. Where does or where has your Free expression shown up in your life?

2. What do you resist or find most off-putting about Free Mamas?

3. Where do you resist this aspect of the Free Mama within yourself?

4. Who's your favorite Free Mama and what do you admire about her?

5. Where can you see parts of her reflected in you?

6. How might your life change from integrating more of your Free expression into your life and being?

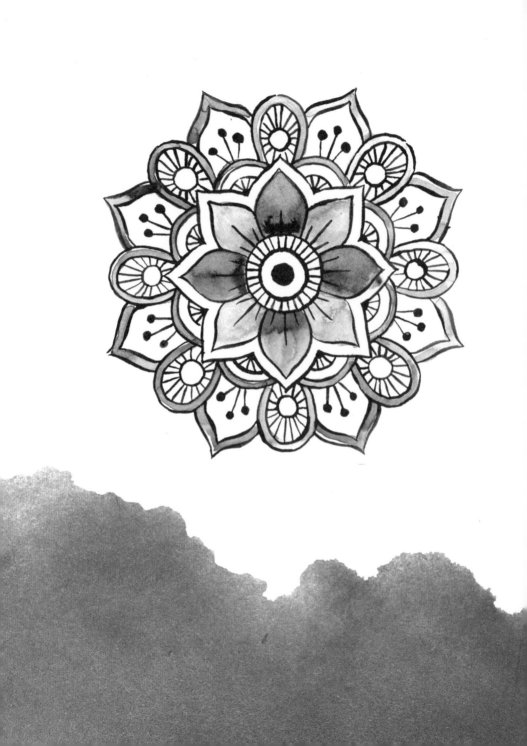

chapter eight

LIVING IN MAMASTE

~~~~~~~~~~~~~~~~~~~~

It fills me with joy when I see my clients make conscious and positive shifts in their lives (whether subtle or dramatic), gather strength as they grow deeper in their self-awareness, and embrace their *whole* self as a mom, wife, partner, daughter, sister, friend, and overall human being. I wish the same for you! I hope that after reading this book, you feel energized and empowered to take what you've learned about yourself and others and step onto your own path toward living in *Mamaste*.

The Greek philosopher Heraclitus wrote, "The only thing that is consistent is change." Surely, nothing demonstrates this more than the all-consuming role of raising children. Year by year, week by week, day to day, even moment to moment, things are constantly changing. You're not only witnessing the incredible milestones of your kids, you're making your own transitions into different phases of motherhood as you grow and evolve right alongside them. You must evolve and adapt to meet each new demand. Evolving and adapting doesn't mean you should or need to become a different person, but it may mean that you need to tap into different expressions that can serve you best at those times. You have everything you need already inside you. Being open and honest with yourself and trusting your own instincts are invaluable tools to help you navigate this complicated journey.

When you feel as if you're experiencing new, uncharted territory, or if you're struggling with a situation or relationship, feel free to retake the quiz on page 27 as way to check in with yourself. Your results may not always be the same, and you'll see right away which expressions you need to integrate or focus on in order to balance things out. You can use this book anytime, when your kids are any age (or, frankly, even before you have kids). You can also use the quiz as a starting point to connect with a partner or friend—it's a helpful way to start a conversation about how you're both feeling and how you can each incorporate the expressions in order to get along more harmoniously.

Annie and Candice, best friends, originally met years ago in the hospital when their daughters were born on the same day. Annie, a true Action Mama, and Candice, who primarily identified as Flow, were instant new-mom buddies, and their dynamic suited them both perfectly. Annie took charge and Candice was happy to go along for the ride. But as the years passed and Candice grew more confident in her role as a mom and friend, she began to tap into her own expression of Action. She started suggesting new places to go on their shared summer vacations, and switched her kids' after-school program—without consulting Annie, something she normally would have done first. This didn't go over well with Annie. She came to me and complained that she felt unappreciated and ignored. I had to remind her that her friendship was evolving along with Candice, and that she needed to allow some space for the shift to happen. I asked, "Could you bring in more of your own expression of Flow or Free to support this new dynamic? How would it feel to loosen the reins by letting some stuff that you are attached to go so you could still enjoy each other's company?"

I checked in with Annie not too long afterward and was thrilled to hear that the two women had worked things out. "We tried Candice's suggestion and ended up loving this amazing eco-resort! We did yoga on the beach together in the mornings—something I definitely would *not* have planned. And even though I miss seeing her with the kids after school, it encouraged me to get to know a few other moms. I guess I don't need to control everything!" she exclaimed. Spoken like a truly balanced Action Mom who has now integrated more Flow into her life.

Remember: You do you. And when it comes to other moms, remember that they're doing *them*. We may express ourselves differently, but we all share the same five expressions! I believe it is absolutely possible for all of us to live authentically and get along without judgment or negativity. It's all about taking that one moment to stop and create a little space to coexist and remind ourselves that we are more alike than different. Focus on the shared goals and the positive outcomes that benefit all people.

There is a wonderful South African philosophy called *ubuntu*, which means, roughly, *A person is a person through other people,* or *I am because you are.* Sound familiar? *The mother in me is the mother in you.* Humanity is not about each of us as individuals, but each of us as individuals sustaining each other and participating in a shared existence together. Think about all the lessons we teach children in their first few years of life—be kind, share, take turns, help clean up—and how quickly those lessons seem to disappear when adults lose their cool. Seeing the world through our kids' eyes is an incredible opportunity to reexamine the choices we make and celebrate our unique personalities for all their strength and beauty.

Action. Flow. Rebel. Vulnerable. Free. What expression are you channeling right now? I am excited for you to own it, use it, honor it, respect it, and see it reflected in others. I wish you a lifetime of harmony and balance, health and happiness, and above all, the courage to always express your authentic truth.

Mamaste.

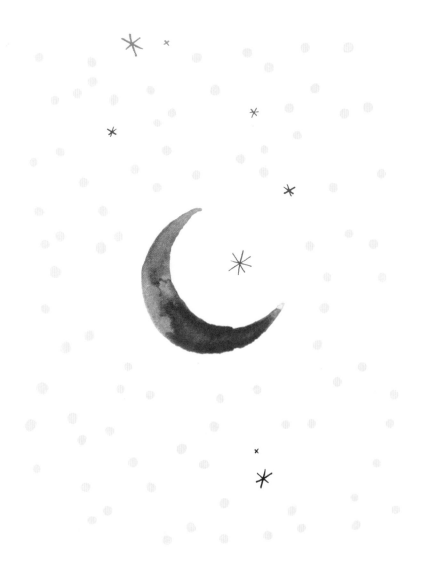

acknowledgments

I want to thank each and every woman I have been so blessed and honored to work with throughout her fertility, pregnancy, birth, and new motherhood journey. My intention behind *Mamaste* is to help many more women find balance and harmony within themselves as well as in the mom world. I would never have been able to write this book and share this wisdom if it weren't for you all. Deep thanks to all of you amazing mamas out there.

Ursula Cary, thank you for saying yes to writing this book with me. Your support, direction, wisdom, and guidance were EVERYTHING! Thanks for putting up with my crazy texts and calls and helping talk me off the ledge when I felt worried or lost with the writing process. I could not have done this without you! I love you, woman!!!

Thank you to Kristin Kosinski for roping me in and keeping me on track while creating structure in a way that worked authentically for me. You helped pull the wisdom and magic out of me and make sense of it on paper. I am forever grateful. You ROCK, lady!!!

Brandi Bowles, you are the best literary agent EVER. Thank you for believing in me and my vision for *Mamaste*. I count my blessings everyday that you are a huge gift in my life! To Rachel Hiles, thank you for seeing the potential in this project.

Camaren Subhiyah, thank you for your amazing edits and making everything flow so easily. You have been a total joy to work with! Designer and illustrator, Cat Grishaver, you are beyond talented! Your vision and artwork helped bring this book to life in such a beautiful way, beyond my wildest dreams! I'm so honored to work with you all and the rest of the incredible team at Chronicle Books.

To my friends and family, thank you for all your love, support, and encouragement. And special thanks to Michele Meiche for being the best soul coach! I wouldn't be the person I am today without your guidance.

xo,

index

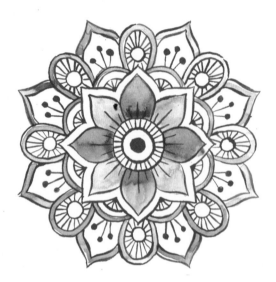